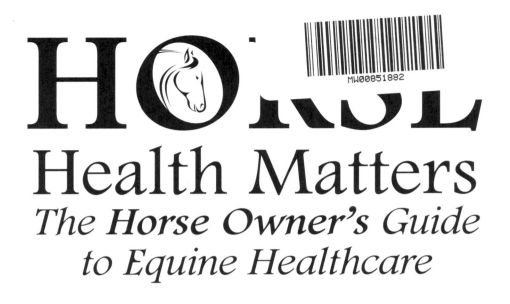

HORSE
Health Matters
The Horse Owner's Guide to Equine Healthcare

Mark Sellers & Flossie Sellers
EquiMed Press

Illustrated by Jo Anna Rissanen

Dedication

To Haley, for bringing the joy of animals into our home.

Published by EquiMed Press, Morgan Hill California

Printed in the United States by Sheridan Books, Inc.
10 9 8 7 6 5 4 3 2 1

Paperback ISBN 978-09-8953-560-1

Table of Contents

Preface

When thinking about this new book on horse health, we wanted to take an approach that is different from the traditional veterinary guides that are usually the first horse health book purchased by the horse owner. The problem with veterinarian guides is that they focus on biological systems and disease, and are more technical than needed for the typical horse owner. Another problem is they often miss covering important topics related to horse handling, behavior and management.

This book takes a fresh approach, addressing the "big picture" topics that you will encounter as you enter the world of horse ownership. These topics are covered in chapters on behavior and training, fitness, nutrition, maintaining a healthy barn and more. Each chapter provides practical and useful advice, and important takeaways that you can immediately act upon to improve your horse's health and safety.

Horses are expensive animals to acquire and maintain. It is wise to understand that the cost of the horse itself is only a minor part of the cost of ownership. Feeding, housing, veterinarian and farrier costs - all add up to a sizeable amount of cash. One priority of this book is to help you reduce your cost of horse ownership by helping you be proactive in preventing diseases, accidents, and other health issues before they result in veterinary bills.

Another priority of this book is to keep you and your horse safe. Horses can be dangerous, mostly because of their weight and strength and core nature. Handling and riding horses is literally an "accident waiting to happen." Your awareness of this potential, along with techniques outlined in this book, can improve your safety and reduce the likelihood of serious injury.

The final and most important priority of this book is to help you get the most out of your horse in terms of enjoyment, and satisfaction. Healthy horses result from caring owners who gain more than they give in their horse-human relationship. This book provides you with a level of understanding that can greatly increase the pleasure that you receive in caring for your horse.

We hope you enjoy this book as much as we enjoyed researching and writing it.

Acknowledgements

Owning and enjoying horses is a group activity. Along with family members or friends, the group includes veterinarians, farriers, feed suppliers, trainers, and often a community at the boarding stable and at shows. Fortunately (and unfortunately), everyone in the group has opinions about what is best for your horse. We start this book by acknowledging all the people that have provided us with advice, both good and bad, always with a well-intentioned attempt to help out.

This book draws most heavily on the many expert contributors to the author's website, http://equimed.com. Their willingness to share their knowledge and expertise plus their love of equines has made this book a classic. Although too many to name individually, their down-to-earth contributions have provided the authors with much of the information that is available in this book.

A special thanks to equine artist Jo Anna Rissanen whose exceptional talent coupled with her personal experiences with equines, veterinarians, farriers has allowed her to show not only the beauty of the horse, but also the complexity of issues of horse health in her illustrations for this book. Indeed, a picture is worth a thousand words when it comes to her rich illustrations.

My mother, Flossie Sellers, is coauthor of this book. In reality, most of the writing and research was done by Flossie, taking the time to learn and explore the ins and outs of horse healthcare. Her diligent effort over the years it took to develop this book are evident in the content quality. Certainly, without her effort, this book would still be a concept existing solely at the back of my mind.

Behind every horse owner are family members and friends that support this expensive habit. My wife, Jacqueline Sellers, grew up a city gal in San Francisco, California. Her support and love, and her willingness to take care of us at horse shows and pitch in at the barn are hugely appreciated. Words truly cannot express my love for her.

Lastly, the reason that our lives have become ingrained within the horse world - our daughter Haley. When we moved to our home in Morgan Hill, California, my then 11 year-old daughter, Haley, decided she wanted to join the local 4-H horse project. Having been an active girl scout, and looking for a change, we decided that the horse project would be a great way for us to connect with our new rural community.

I'm sure that you, good reader, have heard or lived a similar story. We bought our first horse; then we needed a horse trailer, so we found an old 2-horse trailer. Of course, we now needed a bigger truck to haul the trailer. What about a barn. Don't forget the tack and lessons. Of course I got tired of walking when Haley took those trail rides, so why not another horse? On and on it went, and continues to go.

Ten years, five horses and six donkeys later - Haley is now studying veterinary medicine at Michigan State with the desire to enter a large animal practice upon graduation. We are naturally proud of her, but in retrospect, our lives have benefited immensely through the trials and tribulations of horse ownership. The wonderful animals have taught us patience, helped us keep in shape, and provided us bumps, bruises and broken bones along the way. Naturally, they deserve to be acknowledged too:

Horses: Moonstone, Wilbur, Chico, Copper, Boo, and Romeo

Donkeys: Chester, Lucy, Sam, Audry, Sicily and Popcorn

Mark Sellers - 2015

Introduction

Owning a horse is an amazing and rewarding experience. For many of us, horse ownership becomes a lifestyle and greatly influences what we do with our leisure time. Caring for a horse is expensive and time consuming and requires a fairly wide range of knowledge. This book will provide you with a comprehensive education about the variety of health care related issues and activities that you will share with your horse.

This book approaches horse healthcare in a unique manner, and is unlike other "veterinarian guides" that are often owned but seldom used by horse owners. This book breaks healthcare into the 10 categories related to health and well-being:

1. **Behavior**

   Why a horse acts the way he does, and how you can take advantage of this knowledge to better and more safely train your horse. This chapter also touches on learning theory and the techniques that you can use to train your own horse.

2. **Dental care**

   Often forgotten, but vitally important to reducing the cost of ownership, routine dental care is required by all horses for a long and comfortable life. Most of us can relate to the pain of dental problems. Don't allow your horse to live life in pain due to poor dental care.

3. **First aid**

   Let's face it, horses in a domestic setting can be marvelously accident prone. You will be the first line of defense when injury occurs, and in most cases, you can take care of it without requiring a vet visit.

4. **Fitness and conditioning**

   Horses need a physical outlet to be mentally and physically healthy. Keeping your horse fit requires a time investment, but results in a more beautiful and safe animal. You will also benefit from the level of activity required to keep your horse fit.

5. **General care**

   This wide ranging topic covers preventative care that you can do to save money and have a more healthy horse. Preventative care include vaccinations, parasite control, and an awareness of basic equine nutrition.

6. **Hoof care**

   All horses require periodic hoof care, fortunately, most horses don't require shoes. Your farrier and veterinarian are the core members of your hoof care team. Learn what a farrier does, and what you can do to keep your horse's hooves healthy.

7. **Healthy barn**

   Make your barn a place that reduces injury, and promotes the best health for your horses. Horses prefer to live outside, but in many situations, this is impossible. This chapter helps you horse-proof your barn, and will keep you, your animals and your barn visitors safer.

8. **Lameness**

   A horse's legs are both their greatest assets and their greatest liabilities. Capable of outrunning or killing most predators, the horse's legs are also amazingly fragile. Your horse will suffer lameness from time to time. Recognize and treat lameness, and understand when veterinary help is required.

9. **Nutrition**

   Many horse owners become enamoured with complicated feeding protocols, including all sorts of supplements to take care of all sorts of conditions. In reality, most horses do best with a forage based diet, with available salt, minerals a fresh water. Learn about the basics in this chapter that you will use every day.

10. **Reproductive care**

    Few of us have breeding as a goal for our horses. Indeed, because of unintentional and intentional but misguided breed- ing by horse owners, there is an abundance of unwanted horses. This chapter will help you decide if breeding your horse is a good idea, and also let you know what modern technologies are available to help you.

You can find entire books that treat each of these subjects in detail, but in general, these books provide much more information than is required by the horse owner. This book is written to fill the gap for both new and experience horse owner who want to gain information about the range of issues that relate to horse health care.

How to use this book

The chapters of this book are arrange alphabetically based on the 10 general topics mentioned above. The chapter order does not imply any sort of priority, and you should use this book to focus on topics that are of highest interest to you.

The General Care chapter is the recommended place to start your exploration of horse healthcare. This chapter focuses on preventative care, and touches on many subjects that are covered in more detail elsewhere in the book. We consider this chapter a "must read" and "read first"! This chapter alone will put you far ahead in providing basic healthcare for your horse.

Related materials

With the help of our publisher, EquiMed Press, we have created a number of short videos that illustrate topics throughout the book. These video and other resources are provided exclusively to book owners who have purchased the book at the http://horse-health-matters.com website. Look for the video icon for the direct URL of the video, or visit: http://horse-health-matters.com/videos for a complete list.

This website also has a list of updated errata for the printed book, along with additional horse health information, and special offers for other books by the authors.

Danger, warning and caution

Working with horses can be dangerous. These animals can be unpredictable, and have formidable potential weapons in the form of teeth and hooves. Horses are massive, and are capable of crushing you, or running over you. Be careful when working with your horse, and never perform any healthcare or training activity if you are unsure of your safety. Rely on healthcare and training professionals to handle and care for your horse if you have any doubt about your safety. In cases of injury or disease, your horse may react to human contact in an unpredictable and unsafe way.

Throughout this book, we have highlighted areas where safety is a concern. Please pay attention to these cautions and warnings, and do not place yourself in harms way.

Danger: Indicates a hazardous situation which, if not avoided, will result in death or serious injury. The signal word "DANGER" is to be limited to the most extreme situations. DANGER should not be used for property damage hazards unless personal injury risk appropriate to these levels is also involved.

Warning: Indicates a hazardous situation which, if not avoided, could result in death or serious injury. WARNING should not be used for property damage hazards unless personal injury risk appropriate to this level is also involved.

Caution: Indicates a hazardous situation which, if not avoided, could result in minor or moderate injury. CAUTION without a safety alert symbol may be used to alert against unsafe practices that can result in property damage only.

Please be careful

The authors and publishers of this book are not responsible if you are injured when caring for your horse, even when following information contained in this book. Please be careful!

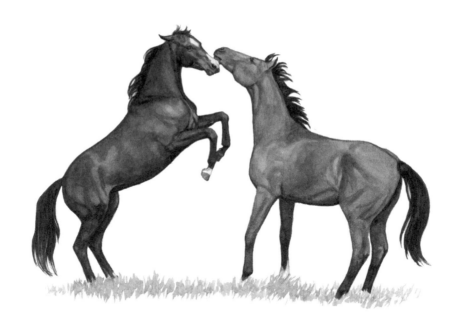

Chapter 1 Behavior

Introduction

This chapter will help you understand why your horse behaves the way he does. You can take advantage of this knowledge for a safer and more rewarding relationship. The horse is unique among "companion" animals. While dogs and cats adapt to living with you in close and cooperative contact, the horse - human relationship is distinctly different. A horse does not adapt to the nature or circumstances of the human. Rather, he simply allows us to adapt to the nature of the horse. Despite, or perhaps because of these differences, the horse-human bond can be powerful and rewarding.

People new to horses often approach a horse like they would a familiar dog. In most cases, the results are mutually inadequate. Dogs are predators and are adapted to a greeting ritual that is high energy and direct. Horses are prey animals. Anything new or unexpected causes the horse's self-preservation instincts to kick-in, causing immediate and sometimes explosive reactions.

Horses generally like to be led. New horse handlers often face the horse and tug helplessly on the halter rope while the animal refuses to budge. Yet, if the handler simply turns in the direction of desired travel and gives a light verbal cue, that same horse follows effortlessly. The key is understanding equine behavior.

Our horses have a simple nature, and very simple needs. We will guide you to a better understanding of horse behavior by showing you how horses perceive their world and how they communicate with each other. You will learn how to take advantage of the core nature of your horse so you can accelerate your training efforts and improve your safety. We will also touch upon some stereotypical behaviors caused by the unnatural environments in which we place our horses!

Evolution

The physical and behavioral evolution of the domesticated horse began in the early Eocene period. As long as 50 million years ago, a small mammal known as Eohippus began browsing on live shoots and the leaves of trees. Scientists have documented this history with a comprehensive collection of fossils tracing the prehistoric animal to the modern horse, *Equus ferus caballus*, that emerged 2.5 to 3.5 million years ago. From the Eohippus, subsequent stages in the evolution of the horse lead to animals with larger bodies, an increased capacity to learn, and other physical refinements, especially regarding the legs and feet. Multiple toes became a single functional toe. Pads became hooves. Bones lengthened and fused to provide support and speed for the larger animal.

Over this same period, changes to the digestive system also occurred allowing the former forest dwellers to successfully occupy open steppes and plains, principally in North America. Durable teeth to chew abrasive grasses, an elongated muzzle for easier reach, and hind-gut fermentation to digest tougher plant material resulted in an animal that was able to thrive.

Eventually, browsing horses crossed back and forth over the land bridge along what is now known as the Bering Straits between North America and Siberia. Then, some 8,000 to 10,000 years ago, the horse followed the

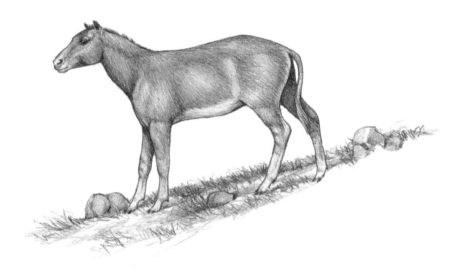

Eohippus
This small and timid browser of the Americas is the distant relative of the modern horse.

mammoth, camel, and other large American mammals into extinction and was reintroduced when Columbus landed the animals in Haiti in 1493. These grazing animals adapted to their habitats by growing larger, developing high crowned teeth, a longer muzzle, changes to the eye structure allowing a wider field of vision, lengthening of limbs and development of hooves to replace their former toes. The brain and loco-motor systems developed specialization capabilities, giving horses mental alertness and the ability to sustain flight and outrun predators.

Survival of the horse in modern times results from its ability to live with and cooperate with humans. First as a work tool and now as a unique companion animal, horses have become integrated into most societies as a valued partner of humans while maintaining the essential characteristics that led to their survival.

How horse behavior links to physical evolution

Behavioral evolution of the horse was closely linked to the physical evolution because of the necessity of survival. The horses that adapted to the environment lived longer than animals that did not adapt.

Along with always being on the alert, early horses learned the general principle of safety in numbers and this led to the development of a strong social hierarchy with built-in protection for the herd. As you observe horses, you will note that they are also naturally wary. This wariness leads to a fear of confined spaces from which they don't have an avenue of escape and, as you will note, any time a horse senses he is being confined to a small space

> **Note**
> Docility vs. performance
>
> Horses maintain their highly reactive nature, in part because breeders prefer animals that are sensitive to physical cues.
>
> Other domesticated livestock, such as cows and chickens, have lost much of their reactive nature through captive breeding.

such as a trailer, alertness, anxiety and a natural instinct to escape will create a challenge for the care taker of the horse.

Watch out for predators

A horse knows instinctively that he has two options when confronted with an unknown threat - flight or fight. Given a threatening situation, the horse's main motivation is to escape and get to a place where he feels safe and free. The horse's natural reluctance to have a saddle or person on his back is related to the fear of a predator gaining control by jumping on its back to bring it down. This instinct is in direct opposition to what most people want to do with their horses which is to jump on and go for a ride. Fortunately, when young horses are trained well, this reluctance can be overcome with patience and reassurance.

Follow the leader

Paradoxically, because the horse needs safety in numbers, this close association can also result in dangerous conflict at times. Nature's solution to this potential problem is to provide a social hierarchy that offers both

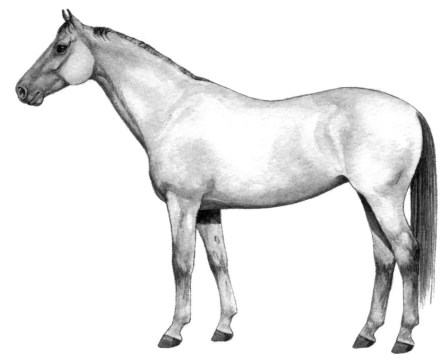

Modern Horse
Large, long-limbed and powerful, the modern horse has prospered because of its utility and beauty.

comfort and leadership to the herd members. Within the hierarchy, the relationship among herd mates is orderly, based on an established dominance with each horse knowing his or her position relative to the others.

In general, the oldest mare leads the band, seeking food and water and safe places to rest. The females within the herd are very social and may spend a lifetime together. Younger animals, including juvenile stallions, are protected by the herd. Conflicts and aggression are minimized as the dominant stallion defends the herd from outside males.

Avoid being trapped

A horse's mental state is closely related to the availability of an escape route. Instinctive fear takes over when the horse feels trapped. This fear can turn into dangerous panic as the horse wants to escape from a potential threat. Despite thousands of years of domestication, the self-preservation instinct toward flight is powerful. Fortunately, horses have the ability to accept and trust humans, and through this trust, the horse can be trained to accept confinement and control. Closely related to a rather claustrophobic nature, horses are very particular and cautious about their legs and feet. A horse will pull its foot away when an attempt is made to pick it up because of this instinctive fear. This is why, we must teach our horse to have his foot lifted from an early age in preparation for farrier care. Also, most horses become fearful and wary when a dog runs around while their hooves are being picked or shoed and they are forced to stand on three legs. This natural wariness exists because dogs are similar to wolves and other historic predators of horses.

From wild to domestic

In short, the historic physical changes in the horse's body and mind have a direct influence on the way domesticated horses see the world and the humans with whom they interact. In times of stress, horses will act from instinct whether it is to strike out or flee. Horses in a domestic setting look for guidance and leadership. It is up to you to take your role as herd leader seriously and act upon it. A delicate balance between trust and respect of authority needs to be established from the beginning with your horses. An undisciplined horse will revert to its natural instinctive behaviors when he feels frightened or threatened. An undisciplined or fearful horse is a potentially dangerous one.

Perception

As a grazing animal that survived for millions of years in the wild, it stands to reason that a horse's senses are more highly developed and more nuanced than those of a human. Good eyesight and a wide range of vision along with exceptional hearing, plus the ability to discern the slightest odor of a predator on the breeze, and the ability to discern the edibility of a plant by a touch of the muzzle and a taste by the tongue meant the difference between life and death for the horse in the wild.

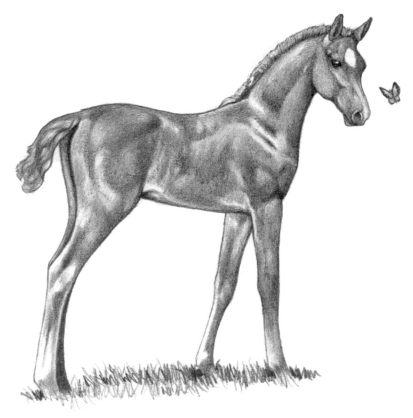

Perception

Horses are very curious and approach novel situations with caution. Fortunately, your horse can become accustomed to scary objects with time and patience.

Eyes and sight

Sight is probably the most important of the equine senses. With eyes on the side of its head, the horse can see almost all around, although a blind zone exists directly behind him and a little in front of his head. Because of these blind spots, it is important not to approach your horse from the rear unless the horse knows you are there, Also, it is important to approach your horse at an angle when approaching from the front.

Although no one knows just how far horses can see, they are known to be able to distinguish patterns at least a hundred yards away and can perceive depth quite well. People who have studied horse's eyes and the way they see tell us that the upper and lower extremes of the horse's eye are for distant vision and the center of the eye focuses on near objects.

Because of the way the horse's eyes are placed, horses need to keep their heads low to focus on objects close beside them. If they are not allowed to keep their heads low and tilt them sideways, they often compensate by skipping sideways to see the object better which may be seen as spooking or shying by an inexperienced rider. Be careful to give your horse his head when approaching scary objects to reduce this skittish behavior.

The horse's eyes convey a wide range of emotions. Horses may be feeling worried, curious, kind, gentle or fearful. Learn to watch your horse's eyes for signals about his emotional state.

A horse is said to have a "Soft Eye" when it is in a gentle and relaxed state of mind. You will notice that your horse begins blinking more as it is processing information or trying to accomplish a new task. A soft eye is a good indicator of the overall nature of the horse. A horse is said to have a "Hard Eye" when it is tense or resistant. The horse will often raise its head, pull back on the lead rope and provide a hard eye when it is being loaded into a trailer. A hard eye is a signal to you to slow down and consider the horse's mental state and the reason for his resistance.

When a horse becomes fearful, and approaches panic, he will open his eyes wide to the extent that you can observe the whites around the margin. This is a signal for you to prepare for a potentially explosive flight response. Immediately retreat from the source of the panic, and do not attempt to force a horse to do anything when he is in a state of approaching panic signaled by the whites of its eyes.

Ears and hearing

An animal that survives by getting a head start on predators necessarily develops a keen sense of hearing. Horses ears are funnel shaped and very mobile. Watch a horse as it reacts to sounds all around. The ear, acting as a funnel for capturing sound and sending it down into the ear canal, swivels and seems to reach toward the sound.

This ability to perceive and process sound quickly and efficiently serves the horse well, although loud, unfamiliar noises can send a horse into flight or a combative attitude if it feels threatened.

Horses are naturally aware and suspicious of movements at distances. They are tuned to capture these sounds and movements long before we do. Paying attention to the horse's ears helps the experienced rider or handler locate the source of concern and be aware of the potential for spooking or bolting.

Amazingly, a soft gentle voice that is calm and confident can work wonders with gaining the cooperation of a horse. With their keen sense of hearing, horses respond well to the sound of the human voice. Keep this idea in mind always and especially when you and your horse are in a noisy or frightening environment.

Nose and smell

Horses have an acute sense of smell and use it to interpret their world in ways that are far beyond the capabilities of a human. The slightest breeze bringing a dangerous scent puts a horse into a flight mode. Horses also relate to their immediate environment through their sense of smell. They greet each other nose to nose and recognize each other by scent and by sight. Mares and foals immediately learn each others scents and can find each other quickly in a crowd of

> ## Tip
> ### Horse greetings
> Observe horses greeting one another and you will notice them smelling each others breath. You may want to copy this greeting behavior by gently breathing into the nose of your horse. Smell his sweet breath too!

horses. Horses come to recognize people in the same way. Notice that recognition when you approach a horse; the horse reaches out his muzzle to take in your scent by sniffing you. Similar to how they greet each other, your horse will smell your breath if permitted to help him identify you.

Muzzle, skin and touch

The equine learns about its environment through its mouth and muzzle as it explores new or different places and people. A mare will reassure her foal with a brush of the muzzle. Horses communicate and scratch each others' itches with their teeth. The horse's muzzle, and lips, signal emotions, needs, and state of mind. The relaxed and contented horse's lips are relaxed. A drooping lower lip indicates a resting or drowsy horse, or a horse that is under sedation from a medical procedure. Curious or playful horses will often extend their lips to explore clothing, hats or pockets of their handlers. Experienced handlers, including farriers, become accustomed to horses probing with their lips, and often ignore this behavior, but generally, it is best to not allow a lipping behavior that may lead to nipping and biting.

Not only are the mouth and muzzle important to the horse's sense of touch, but the skin is also. Although horse skin is believed to be tough, it has many nerve endings and can sense the tiniest fly landing on the horse's rump. An astute horse owner knows the value of a rub on the horse's shoulder or a vigorous message over a tense muscle. Your touch tells your horse, "Hey, I'm your friend," and, in many cases, the horse will return the compliment with a touch or a look that speaks volumes.

> **Tip**
> ## A calming touch
>
> Agitated or fearful horses can be calmed with physical contact. Horses do not like to be patted or slapped, but they do respond to smooth stroking or rubbing on the shoulders, poll area and the croup.

Yes, a horse's senses are a determining factor in his behavior. Knowing the significance of your horse's senses and the accompanying signals along with how they work in relationship to their environment will enable you to be more "in tune" with your horse.

Language

Equines "converse" with each other all the time. They constantly use

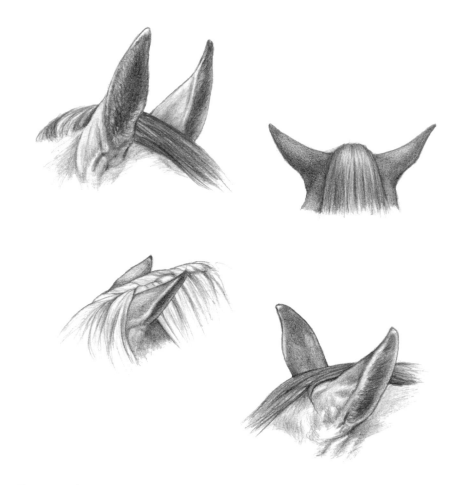

Expressive ears

Observing your horse's ears can tell you much about their mental state. Clockwise from upper left - Alert, Resting, Attentive, and Angry of Fearful.

facial, vocal and body signals to communicate with each other. Understanding the basics of equine language is extremely important in accurately assessing what is happening with your horse and how it perceives you and the world around it.

Equine language intersects closely with the senses: hearing, sight, smells, touch, and taste. Based on use of their senses, horses then react to their perceptions through vocal and physical acts that convey. Your horse is a master at reading body language, how you carry yourself and move around your horse is important in removing fear and establishing the important leadership role.

Reading your horse's body language
Ears

Highly expressive, and easily visible to a mounted rider or while on the ground, a horse's ears are excellent communicators of his mental state at any given instance.

The horse's ears constantly give clues about where the horse's attention is focused and how he is interpreting what is happening.

Different positions of the ears can enable the alert observer to determine the general attitude of the horse. A horse on alert lifts its neck and focuses both ears and eyes in the direction of a perceived threat. If the ears are pricked forward, the horse is giving extreme attention in that direction. Ears to the side show the attention to be in that direction. Ears flat back usually show anger or fear, while both ears drooping show relaxation and drowsiness. A relaxed horse's ears are held at approximately 45 degrees from the poll and point slightly down and forward. This is a natural and comfortable state, observed when horses are resting or feeling safe and secure.

> ## Note
> ### Masters of body language
> Horses are keenly observant of body language, and use it to establish dominance within the herd. Trainers learn to use their body language as an important tool in gaining respect and communicating with the horse.

When a horse is working or is occupied with a specific task, the ears work independently, with each focusing on a different sound or cue. The attentive ear action is observed in horses that are being trained or handled, and this signals that the horse is paying attention to whatever activity they are performing. Trainers look for this type of ear language as a signal that the horse is engaged in the training activity.

An aggressive or angry horse lays its ears back and lowers its head as a threat warning. The threat gesture is very common in groups of horses as they establish the herd hierarchy. Subordinate horses move away from dominant horses when presented with the pinned ears. Pinned ears directed at a human indicate a lack of respect that may lead to aggression.

Tail

The tail is used as a visual signal of the horse's emotional state. When happy and playful, horses will "flag" their tails, lifting them and swishing them as they run and play. In a natural setting where mares are part of a harem, the mares will "high-tail" and "flag" their tails to attract the stallion, often while presenting a lowered head showing submission.

Horses show annoyance by swishing and flipping their tails. The annoyance may be caused by persistent flies, irritation with the closeness of a subordinate horse, frustration due to isolation. A horse in training or at a show may exhibit resistance when being asked to perform a difficult task, such as changing leads at a slow gait. A seasoned rider listens to the tail swish as an indicator that resistance is increasing.

Head and neck

Head and neck set are important in recognizing the horse's attitude in relationship to what is happening. We have all seen horses startled by movement on the horizon. In order to gain a better view, an fearful or anxious horse will elevate his head, and focus ears and eyes in the direction of the feared object.

During rest, the horse will lower his head to the level of his withers. A lowered head is also a signal from stallions to mares as the stallion essentially herds his harem of mares with a lowered head and pinned ears. A mare in estrus will also lower her head to signal receptiveness to the stallion.

Legs

Horses that are nervous or fearful will dance around. This fearful state may result in a horse attempting to escape so it is incumbent on the handler to divert the horse's attention and calm it with a gentle soothing voice.

A horse will often paw the ground as a result of frustration. Leaving a horse tied for a long period of time, especially a hungry or thirsty horse, will often result in pawing the ground around the tie post. Foot stamping is often a result of mild irritation due to flies, especially biting flies.

A horse that is threatened may lift his hind leg as a signal before kicking. This warning sign is important to recognize as the threat may be followed by a dangerous kick. Horses that swing their hips in the direction of a person and threaten to kick should be retrained by a skilled professional.

A resting horse will often "cock" a back leg, resting it on the tip of the hoof. This is normal for the horse, and is a sign that the horse is comfortable and resting.

Understanding to your horse's voice

Horses have a wide range of vocal signals which they have used to their advantage down through history. Following are some of the important vocal signals horses use:

- Neigh: contact or recognition
- Nickers: depends on relationship: a stallion's courtship nicker; maternal nicker of mare to foal; friendship nicker to human with food
- Squeal: very close contact, especially sexual
- Snort: alarm, challenge excitement
- Screams and roars: extreme emotional state, rage, fear. If a horse screams or roars at you, get out of the way. It really means to hurt you. (Very rare)
- Grunts: effort, fighting, jumping; in cases of pain or colic, not an intentional signal
- High blowing noise made in false nostril: sign of pleasure especially when cantering
- Nose blowing or clearing: relaxed, happy with environment or work

By being alert to your horse's facial, vocal and body language signals, understanding and communicating with your horse will take on new and effective dimensions.

Body signals can give you invaluable information about your horse and his perception of what is happening. If a horse is striking out, head tossing, bucking or rearing, you immediately know that the animal is defiant, aggressive, frustrated or confused. If these actions occur with a rider in the saddle, it means the horse isn't listening, is receiving mixed signals, or simply is not willing to cooperate.

Danger
Flight vs. fight

Horses react and take flight much quicker than you can respond. Combining a huge mass with lightning reactions can be lethal for anyone in the flight path. NEVER stand directly in front of your horse and ALWAYS be aware of potential sources that may spook your horse.

As you approach your horse each time, make a mental note of whether his body and muscles are tensed or relaxed. Look at the tail, the neck and withers, and their positions in relationship to the rest of the body. Observe the ears and how the horse is breathing. Is he relaxed, labored, or holding his breath? By looking at the horse's stance and noting body, facial and vocal signals, you will gain insight into your horse's state of mind.

The horse as a herd animal

Horses are highly social herd animals that prefer to live in a group. In times of stress, whether from predators or extreme weather, the center of the herd is the safest because it offers the most protection from the elements and is further away from predators than any other part. Because of this, punishment of misbehaving members is sometimes delivered in the form of expulsion from the herd, either temporarily or sometimes permanently.

Feral and wild horse herds are usually made up of several separate small bands that share a given territory. Often a dominant mare leads the herd which contains additional mares, their foals, and immature horses of both sexes. There is usually a single "herd" or "lead" stallion, though occasionally a few less-dominant males may remain on the fringes of the group. A linear dominance hierarchy exists in any herd. The horses establish a "pecking order" for the purpose of determining which herd member directs the behavior of others by eating and drinking first and leading the herd as it moves across the landscape. Any fights for dominance are normally brief, and sometimes merely displaying dominant gestures without physical contact is enough.

Horses and humans

Humans are usually viewed by wild horses as potential predators. However, horses are also innately curious and may investigate any creature that is interesting but not threatening. Any domesticated horse with some experience of humans usually views people as generally harmless objects of curiosity worth at least minor notice, especially if they know that humans may bring food or treats.

Rarely will any domestic horse become truly vicious unless it has been spoiled or abused by humans, although many stallions are naturally aggressive with dominant behaviors that require strong, knowledgeable handlers.

The horse and human partnership

The ability of humans to work in cooperation with the horse is based on both the natural curiosity of the horse and the strong social bonds that horses have with each other. Horses do not like to be separated from their herd because to be alone is to be exposed to predators on all sides. Also, in a herd, less dominant horses tend to gravitate toward the most mature and confident members.

Many horse training principles are based on having the horse accept a human as the dominant herd member. Ideally this is not done by force, but by the horse developing trust in the ability of the human and confidence that the human will be a responsible herd leader.

This willingness to consider new things can also be used by a human trainer to adapt the horse's behavior to an extraordinary range of activities that are well outside the range of instinctive horse behavior, including acts considered naturally dangerous by the average horse such as bullfighting, jumping off cliffs, diving into water, or working on a movie set.

Horses are also adapted to covering large amounts of territory and must have a certain boldness to do so. A horse that is afraid more than necessary will expend energy needlessly and then may not be able to escape when a threat is real. Therefore, horses have the ability to check out the unusual and not immediately flee from something that is merely different, and, with patience, this energy and boldness can be harnessed for effective achievements in training.

Testing boundaries

Horses have to be conditioned to the fact that some normal herd behavior is inappropriate around humans. For example, biting and "shadow boxing" activities such as rearing, or striking that is common play among young horses, colts in particular, can be injurious or fatal to people. Other instinctive traits, such as running away when frightened, bucking off anything that lands on a horse's back, or never entering a small enclosed area, also have to be overcome through patient, consistent training.

Horse have been compared to three-year-old children by one horse expert. Like three-year-old children, they have relatively short attention spans, usually accept what they are taught, and can be forgiving shortly after having been called out because of misbehavior. Most horses will still test boundaries over and over, at least mildly, and some horses with dominant personalities will openly challenge a weak or inexperienced handler.

For example, if handled with incompetence or abuse, a horse may ignore its training and attempt to nip, bite, kick, refuse to be led, or try other ways to challenge human dominance. Without consistent handling, some horses, especially young ones, will revert to untrained ways. However, due to their good memory, horses with consistent training from trustworthy handlers often retain what they have learned, even after a gap of many years. When it comes to behavior, the horse may be summed up as a social, grazing, prey species. Many of the attributes we find in the horse and label as problems are not failings but rather the result of a species that has successfully adapted to its natural environment. For that, we as horse owners should be grateful!

In addition, although horses may prefer the company of other horses, they can accept a human handler and with proper training recognize the human as a dominant member of their "herd" where recognition of important inherited behavioral traits by the handler are put to their best use. This is why a horse owner needs to be well educated in the ways of the horse.

Eating and horse behavior

The way the horse eats is an integral part of horse behavior. Since the horse is an herbivore, it is predictable that much of the behavior is related to the consumption of forages and the use of his hooves to flee or fight when threatened during the foraging process. Behavior has direct effects on consumption patterns, feed availability and the selection of feeds. In the wild, horses devote more time to eating than to any other behavioral activity. In the wild, a number of factors affect the horse's grazing pattern. The location of water, for example, can have an important effect on grazing patterns. In arid zones, the water source is the center of grazing activity and the primary determinant of the grazing area. The area near the water may become overgrazed, even damaged and eroded, because of the influence of the water source on grazing pattern.

Social factors, such as the development of a home or territorial area can inhibit movement of horses on large ranges. The social rank of the horses can determine which horses obtain the choicest grazing sites or best access to supplemental feed or water. These social behaviors carry over into the life of the domesticated horse and horse owners with several horses need to take this into account to make sure that all horses receive the feed and water they need.

Stereotypies

If you have been fortunate enough to see horses in their natural habitat, you appreciate the many ways a horse has had to adapt in the transition from the wild to the domesticated state.

Although horses in their natural habitat faced daunting situations at times, the safety and socialization of the herd helped wild horses to

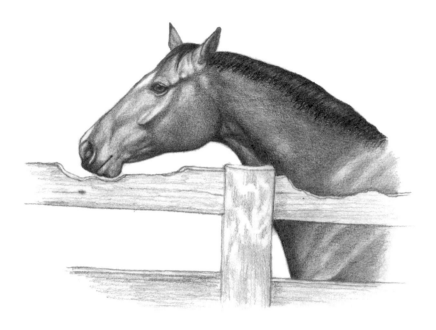

Barn vices

Often caused by boredom, frustration, chronic pain or other maladies, barn vices include obsessive compulsive behaviors called stereotypies.

adapt to their surroundings in such a way that they were kept busy and had plenty of exercise which contributed greatly to their overall health.

With domestication came an unnatural physical setting for the horse that is more isolated, controlled, and often characterized by feed consumption that is radically different from the natural horse environment. Equine science blames these environmental changes as contributors to various obsessive-compulsive behaviors that are not observed in a natural environment.

What research tells us about stereotypies

Currently, "stereotypic behavior" is the preferred term for behaviors that are often referred to as stable vices. Stereotypies are a concern for horse owners because of the damage the horse can do both to itself and

19

to its environment. Although stereotypies are seen by many researchers and horsemen as safety valves that allow a horse to survive stress without becoming neurotic, the preference is to avoid these behaviors because of the damage they inflict on the horse and its environment.

Dr. Georgia Mason is given credit for the classic definition of stereotypies: "Any repetitive behavior performed with no obviously discernible function."

Simple attempts to curb or stop the behaviors may cause more damage than the stereotypy itself. Development of a stereotypy in most cases acts as a warning that the horse is in a frustrating environment and needs to release pressure. The movements and actions involved in the particular stereotypy help the horse to do so.

Factors that play a role in stereotypic behaviors

Housing, management, social contact among horses, proper nutrition, sufficient exercise, physical comfort, and weaning methods are seen as influential factors in the development of stereotypic behaviors, although breed and behavior of the sire and dam may, in some cases, be an influence.

Researchers and horsemen agree that maximizing the horse's welfare is the most effective way of preventing stereotypic behaviors.

The best plan of action is to determine the specific cause or causes of the behavior and then address those causes by removing them or mitigating the effects they have on the horse. In most cases, this results in a reduction of the behavior, but does not result in elimination.

Three kinds of stereotypies

In general, stereotypies fall into three groups: oral; locomotion; and other. Oral stereotypies are usually identified as cribbing or wind sucking, wood chewing, bed eating, dirt eating or coprophagy, and mane and tail chewing. Locomotion stereotypies include stall walking, weaving, circling, pawing or digging, stall kicking, and head shaking. Other kinds of stereotypies are not well defined and usually encompass natural horse behavior that becomes problematic when it becomes repetitive such as bucking every time the horse is saddled or rearing repeatedly when attempts are made to catch him.

Oral stereotypies

Oral stereotypies are those repetitious movements the horse makes where the mouth and muzzle are involved such as cribbing or wind sucking.

Research indicates that feeding two bulk meals a day with nothing to nibble on for many hours causes some horses to develop stereotypies involving their lips and mouth.

Cribbing occurs when a horse grasps an object with its teeth, flexes its neck, then pulls back with its teeth while exhibiting a characteristic grunt. Some research indicates that the horse receives an euphoric feeling or a sense of well-being from these actions. Unfortunately, cribbing can lead to weight loss, colic, and excessive tooth wear. Causes of cribbing are usually thought to be boredom, confinement, and lack of exercise.

Wind sucking is similar to cribbing except that the horse does not necessarily bite down on an object. He flexes the neck and sucks air down into its lungs and/or stomach with a distinctive grunt

> ## Note
> ### Cribbing collars
> Cribbing collars are used to stop the cribbing behavior. They work by causing pain when the horse attempts to crib. Most equine behaviorists agree that cribbing collars are cruel, and should not be used.

after the inhalation of the air. This behavior becomes compulsive, and if allowed to continue over a period of time, may lead to malnutrition, weight loss, and colic. Excess confinement and lack of exercise resulting in boredom are considered the main causes of wind sucking.

Although wood chewing is not considered a stereotypy by some researchers, wood chewing is a common occurrence in horses that spend most of their time in stables and are given limited opportunities for foraging in pastures where long-stemmed vegetation is available. Researchers have documented that a horse or pony can eat up to two pounds of wood daily, leading to damaged stalls, fences, and feeders. Once this behavior becomes compulsive and repetitive, it may be considered a stereotypy. Ingestion of slivered wood sometimes results in gastrointestinal irritation or obstructions. Often, simple management changes that include providing horses with plenty of roughage and adequate socialization with other horses, especially in a pasture setting, will help stop this behavior.

Research shows that the more time a horse spends eating, the less likely the horse is to engage in wood chewing. Lack of exercise leading to the need for a release of nervous energy is often seen as a factor in wood chewing. Reducing tension, eliminating boredom, providing adequate exercise, and furnishing feed with a good amount of roughage often result in the elimination of wood chewing.

Changes in management of the horse's daily activities that allow plenty of exercise and socialization, plus the addition of either more foraging time or coarser hay often deter this behavior.

Locomotion stereotypies

Locomotion stereotypies rarely occur in horses living in their natural environments where a wide range of active behaviors occur. But in more confined environments, repetitive behaviors involving locomotion are seen as abnormal and indicative of welfare problems for the horse displaying them.

Stall walking by stabled horses is a rather common occurrence and is usually the result of being confined in a small area, often a box stall, with insufficient exercise. In stall walking, the horse moves around the perimeter of the stall, eventually wearing down the flooring. In some cases, the horse walks slowly, but in other cases, the walking is rapid and the horse appears agitated, often defecating and flicking the ears as it walks aggressively around the stall. Not only is this behavior destructive to the flooring of the stall, but it can also result in hoof and limb problems.

When stall walking takes up much of the horse's time and attention, it can lead to dehydration and loss of weight resulting from lack of interest in eating and drinking.

Weaving is evidenced by the horse rocking back and forth repetitively while standing in place. Animals that have a tendency to be nervous or those that are confined to their stalls for long periods of time without contact with other horses are prone to weaving. Uneven hoof wear and lameness are common occurrences when a horse engages in weaving behavior. In addition, the horse may lose weight and become dehydrated if it engages in this activity to the exclusion of eating and drinking properly. Some research shows that weaving increases with aging of the horse, especially if the horse tends to be distressed or nervous.

Circling is similar to stall walking in that the horse circles around the stall compulsively, either slowly or in an agitated fashion, depending on the temperament of the horse and the amount of energy expended. Weight loss and lameness often become components of a circling stereotypy.

> ## Note
> ### Do horses learn from one another?
> Common barnyard folklore includes the belief that stereotypic behaviors, such as cribbing, can be learned by one horse from another. This often leads to isolation of the affected animal that may exacerbate the problem. In reality, the environment is believed to play a much larger role in the development of these behaviors and mimicry has not been established as a cause.

Pawing on the part of a horse has a number of meanings and uses. When pawing develops the repetitiveness of a stereotypy, it often reflects the horse's frustration or impatience with its environment and may be done with such a fervor that the horse seems unaware of its surroundings and becomes totally engrossed in the pawing action. The pawing may take place in the stall, the trailer, or the paddock. The pawing leads to digging and can create deep holes depending on the surface where the horse is pawing. Pawing can result in abnormal hoof or shoe wear or to loss of shoes, and can lead to lameness and weight loss.

Stall kicking can be a vicious stereotypy depending on the energy level of the horse. Little anecdotal evidence supports the idea that most stereotypies are mimicked or copied from other horses; however, stall kicking is an exception, possibly because it may become a means of communication among horses. Repeated stall kicking damages the horse's hooves and limbs and can cause serious injury. In addition, stall walls and doors are damaged and need constant repairs. As with other locomotion stereotypies, research shows that increased exercise and less confinement and more pasture time will decrease the amount of time a horse spends kicking at stall walls and doors.

Some head shaking is common for most horses and may be caused by a variety of factors, such as eye, ear, or tack problems, allergies, sensitivity to light, insects, and other irritants. When the horse's head shaking becomes a stereotypy, it usually begins as a response to stress and occurs in a repetitive fashion on a regular basis. In fact, careful observation of the horse may show that the repeated head shaking has an almost drug-like effect on the horse, since the behavior triggers the release of endorphins in the brain, causing the animal to feel better. If the head shaking takes place at events or while being ridden, it can affect performance. If it occurs only while the horse is in the stall, it is an indication of boredom and lack of sufficient socialization with other horses. In some cases, head shaking occurs only with certain types of bits or tack, and if this is the case, it may be the result of discomfort, and once the discomfort is alleviated, the behavior stops.

> ## Note
> ### The five freedoms
>
> Animal welfare results by providing for the five freedoms required by all animals in captivity:
>
> 1. Freedom from thirst, hunger and malnutrition
> 2. Freedom from physical and thermal discomfort
> 3. Freedom from pain, injury and diseases
> 4. Freedom to express most patterns of normal behavior
> 5. Freedom from fear and distress
>
> Pay special attention to number 4 - horses are social animals and do best when able to interact with each other in an outdoor setting, such as a pasture or large turnout.

Other stereotypies

"Other" stereotypies are not as well-defined as oral and locomotive stereotypies and usually encompass natural horse behavior carried to the point that it becomes problematic, such as when a horse consistently bucks, shows signs of barn sour, or prances instead of standing still. Whether these are true stereotypies is questionable since they are not repetitive behaviors engaged in for an extended period of time. In many cases, they are bad habits picked up by the horse as a result of poor training or interactions with people and other horses.

Preventing stereotypic behaviors

The key to preventing horses from developing stereotypic behaviors is to reduce conditions that lead to stereotypies in the first place. Research points to horse welfare as the key to the prevention of stereotypies. Chief factors you need to consider in caring for your horse include housing for comfort and socialization, feeding to encourage grazing behaviors, and exercise for physical and mental well-being.

Housing

Stabling horses together in freely associating groups or with family groups allows the contact necessary to prevent the development of stereotypic behaviors. Horses that interact with each other are able to hear, touch, smell and interact with each other frequently and is considered one of the most healthy ways for horses to live. Owners should provide as much visual stimulation as possible with windows in stalls and a clear view of other horses if a horse is restricted to the stall for much of the day. Break-proof mirrors and appropriate lighting also may be useful in providing stimulation for the horse.

If your horse is usually isolated from other animals, consider providing a companion animal. A goat, chickens, a donkey--any animal that provides diversion and company, but that won't be stepped on or escape from the stable, can work as a companion for your horse. For some horse owners, an investment in stable toys pays off with hours of engaged activity for their horses. Although the jury is still out on whether or not stable toys reduce incidents of stereotypic behavior, anything that enriches a horse's environment should be considered.

Feeding

Horses naturally prefer to graze as opposed to bulk meals twice a day. Many horses eat their feed in a relatively short time leaving them little to do for hours on end. These structured, relatively brief feedings do not meet the horse's instinctive urge to forage for food. When horses are fed mostly concentrated feed in quantities larger than the amount needed for the work they do, they tend to develop active stereotypies, possibly as a way to work off the energy content of the feed. Highly concentrated feeds also have less roughage than regular hay and feed which reduces the volume and the time a horse spends eating it.

Providing plenty of hay throughout the day when a horse is confined to a stall for long periods of time can be helpful in providing a "grazing" experience. Automatic feeders are on the market that save both time and effort in making a more natural feeding schedule available for your horse. Having to tug hay out of a hay net over a period of time will also provide the horse with actions similar to foraging, as well as lengthen feeding time. Feeding balls that dribble out small amounts of feed and can be pushed around keep the horse engaged and having to "forage" for feed may be helpful in keeping your horse occupied.

Consider free choice feeding as it most closely emulates natural horse behavior. But be aware that the type and variety of feeds must be nutritionally correct for a free choice situation. Free choice Feed must not provide excessive calories, starch or sugars. See Chapter 9 - Nutrition for more information on free choice feeding.

Always make sure that your horse has an adequate diet including plenty of roughage, a salt lick and supplements where necessary along with feed that provides plenty of chewing.

Exercise

The horse owner that makes sure a horse receives sufficient exercise is rewarded with better behavior. Although a minimum of 30 minutes a day is recommended, a couple of hours are better for many horses. If you are not available to ride your horse or exercise him, hire a neighbor or another interested and responsible person to ride or longe the horse for you.

Give your horse as much turn-out time as possible even in cold weather. If your horse has access to a pasture, this can be the best of all worlds for the horse since it can provide stimulation, exercise, grazing opportunities and socialization either with other horses or with people.

Stereotypic behaviors affect a horse's usefulness, dependability and health. Once established these bad habits are difficult to eliminate and may lead to physiological problems. Many stereotypic behaviors are dangerous to the horse and handler and destructive to property, as well as being genuine nuisances in the barn, stable and arena.

Horse welfare

Research shows that horses that engage in stereotypies show fewer physiological signs of stress than horses that are obviously stressed, but don't engage in stereotypic behaviors. Be wary of claims for devices or training techniques that claim to eliminate stereotypic behaviors. These devices (e.g. cribbing collars) and training techniques are not considered effective, and may actually increase the stress that contributes to negative behaviors.

Training

Every time you interact with your horse, be it feeding, catching, walking, loading, riding, washing, you are training your horse. If you keep this in mind and use your understanding of horse behavior, not only will you be safer, but your horse will learn quicker. Equine researcher J. Hausberger offers an important insight - "Just because you don't intend to teach a horse something doesn't mean that you won't; and just because you are not aware of having taught a horse something doesn't mean you didn't."

Popular "methods"

Horses can easily be trained by the horse owner who is dedicated to learning some basic techniques. These techniques are often packaged into specific "methods" that are provided via DVD or online training by popular horse clinicians. These packages are beneficial to the horse owner, and generally provide sound training techniques in a manner that is easy to understand and easy to use. Most of these products deal with gaining respect through ground-working your horse.

From ground to mounted training

Moving beyond groundwork to mounted training requires the physical coordination, balance and skill of an experienced rider/trainer. For safety and effectiveness, training of young untrained horses is best left to a specialized professional. The first experiences under saddle are important to the young horse that needs to build security and confidence in the rider. An inexperienced horse owner cannot provide the level of security and confidence that is required during the early stages of training.

> ## Danger
> ### Mounted training
>
> For a pray animal such as a horse, having any other animal (such as a human) get on his back can cause some powerful and dangerous reactions. Early mounted work on an untrained horse of any age can be extremely dangerous.

For more mature horses, the average horse owner can be very effective in advancing the level of training. Understanding the basics of horse training via book study should be accompanied by working with a professional trainer for a period to develop the muscle memory and balance that allows your horse to develop trust and confidence.

Training using learning theory

Regardless of the training level of your horse and your own personal experience, understanding these rules that leverage our understanding of basic horse behavior will be key to having a better trained horse:

- Start by gaining respect
- Understand pressure/release
- Train consistently
- Keep training session short
- Use repetition

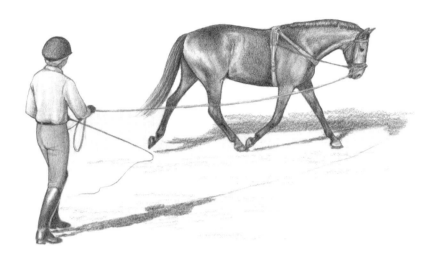

Longeing

Classical horse training incorporates longeing to teach your horse vocal commands, and pressure/release. It also builds your horse's strength and flexibility.

- Use reinforcement
- Know when to quit

Start by gaining respect

Horses love to follow a leader. Your first goal in training your horse is to establish your role as leader. Once accomplished, you will be safer and your horse will be most willing to cooperate. Horses can sense your anxiety or fear, so it is very important to move slowly, and to be calm and deliberate. Avoid any fast movement of your hands, especially around the horse's head. Do not be tentative with your movements. Act like you know what you are doing (even though you may not)!

The first activity for gaining respect is to be able to catch, halter and lead your horse. This may require patience if your horse has not been trained properly.

Catching and leading

After catching and haltering, take your horse for a walk around your pasture or barn. Your control of the horse's movements is an important factor in being recognized as a leader. Do not let the horse push or pull you. Shorten your halter rope to gain control of the head, and walk forward always looking where you want to go and never looking at your horse.

Set a destination goal and lead your horse to the goal. Turn and pat your horse on the shoulder and give him a treat. Apply pressure to the lead rope as needed to begin movement. As soon as movement begins, release all lead rope pressure.

Training your horse "in-hand" is an important part of training. Go to a local horse show and observe a showmanship class. These classes show how a horse and handler work together, in-hand, to perform complex patterns with absolute obedience and control

Longeing and Round Penning

Longeing and round penning are methods used by horse trainers to gain respect. These are natural extensions of controlling the movement of your horse that you began with catching and leading. The key with longeing is that you are maintaining physical contact and control, this time at a distance.

The tools used in longeing are very simple and should be some of the first training equipment investments that you make. In addition to your halter, you will need a longe rope and longe whip and optionally, a good pair of gloves. Our recommended longe rope is easy on the hands, easy to coil, and is an extremely strong 25 foot rolled cotton longe line.

A longe whip needs to be long enough to motivate your horse while longeing. These whips are generally 10 feet long, including handle and whip. Do not use a short carriage whip or think that you can use the end of the rope as these will prove frustrating and ineffective.

The best method of learning to longe your horse is to observe best practices by an expert, and then emulate and practice. Horse Health Matters has produced a short instructional video that will help you get started with longeing your horse.

Round penning is similar to longeing, but the horse is constrained within a circular arena (called a round pen) approximately 50 feet in diameter. A longe line can be used, but as you progress, you should allow the horse to run free. The round pen is a logical step after longeing to encourage your horse to listen to your voice commands, and to be under control of your body and vocal commands.

> ## Note
> ### The importance of timing
> Horses learn by associating the removal of pressure with the correct behavior. The association relies on an almost instantaneous release when the behavior is performed. When riding, always practice lightness, and lightening quick removal of pressure when your horse performs as asked.

Leading, longeing and round penning work to establish your leadership and teaches your horse to respond to pressure coming from a rope, your body language and your voice. To be effective it is very important that you establish and use cues consistently in all training activities.

Most horse trainers establish and use commands that communicate the following controls while leading, longeing or round penning:

- "Whoa" or "ho" to stop
- Cluck sound to move forward or accelerate
- Kiss sound to lope
- "Easy" or "whup" or "hmm" to slow down
- "Back" to back

Only use these words or sounds when training, and never use "Whoa" to slow down. This command should only be used to stop. Learn to give the verbal command once, and then use rope, whip or rein pressure to enforce the command. Giving the command over and over is counter productive and confusing to the horse.

Mounted work

Training respect and control while mounted has many advantages, and some distinct disadvantages. The close contact of your body and legs provide a myriad of cues that can range from subtle to aggressive. The control of the head is improved with opposing reins and a bit placed within the horse's sensitive mouth.

Disadvantages relate to the skill of the rider. Balance may be problematic for the new rider, and inappropriate cues or cue timing can also confuse or frustrate a horse. Also, a fear factor may stiffen the rider, and communicate fear to the horse which is always something to be avoided.

Understanding pressure/release

Horses are finely tuned to a pressure/release method of training. Virtually all modern trainers make use of directed pressure as the means of "asking" for a behavior, followed by a rapid release of pressure when the behavior is accomplished. As a refinement over time, the application and release of the pressure becomes quicker and softer, with an ultimate goal of being as light and soft as is required to accomplish a task.

You have already been using pressure release when you starting haltering and walking your horse. You applied pressure to the lead rope, causing slight discomfort in your horse, and as the horse took his first step forward you released the pressure. Now, when you halter and lead your horse, work to make the pressure (pulling on the rope) followed by a very quick release when the horse moves forward. In short order, you will simply need to lean forward and the horse will walk with you, and stop and your horse will stop by your side as if by magic.

When longeing, you apply pressure by pulling the rope attached to the halter, and also apply pressure by moving your whip. When you started, you probably felt constant pressure on the lead rope as your horse leaned on the rope. After awhile, you will notice that the pressure from the horse pulling becomes less and less. The horse is LEARNING to give to the pressure. You probably also needed to use the whip more when starting to maintain your horse's speed. Over time, the horse learns to avoid whip pressure by maintaining his pace.

In round penning, you lose the physical connection to the horse, and rely on verbal, body language, enforced with the longe whip. If you consistently use the verbal commands, you will quickly be able to exact more and more control with lighter and lighter commands.

As you move from ground work to mounted work, you have a lot more control and responsibility to use pressure and release in a consistent manner. Again, it is critical to avoid confusion. Keep you training sessions focused on only a single response at a time. For example, don't combine a stop with a rollback until your stops are reliable and solid, and your horse has an understanding of rolling back, trained separately. Lastly, make your queues clear and consistent. Each queue should elicit a single response.

Train consistently

When a young horse is trained, it is traditional that he is ridden every day for one or two months. These first 60 rides are critical to establish respect and confidence by the young horse for the rider. During this training, the green-horse trainer will spend only a few rides inside a round pen or arena, and focus on riding the young colt or filly outdoors where it can experience novel conditions and learn to trust the rider.

Training the green horse is a highly dangerous specialty and should be left to a person that has the skill and knowledge to take the green horse and turn it into a "started" horse.

After the horse is "started" he knows the basics and is ready to continue basic training focused more on the intended use of the horse. Arena riding, Eventing, trail riding, ranching - most horses specialize in the uses that are attractive to the rider.

Horses in professional training are normally ridden one hour per day, five days a week. This is the commitment level it takes to produce a horse that can effectively compete in horse shows or athletic competitions.

For the typical horse owner, training and riding may only be practical once or twice a week. This is considered a maintenance level of riding, and benefits both horse and trainer by consistently reinforcing basic training. It also maintains a certain level of condition and a physical release of energy that your horse needs.

Keep training sessions short

Horses are emotionally comparable to three year old children. They learn best from consistent and enforced activities, that are repeated many times. Young horses are easily distracted. Observe their ears, eyes and head position during training sessions, and it appears that they are focused on everything but you, the trainer.

Professional trainers learn that a horse can effectively concentrate and expend the necessary energy for a relatively short period of time before their ability to learn and perform degrades. It is generally accepted that intense training sessions should be limited to one-half hour. With proper warm-up and cool-down, the entire mounted time should be around one hour. Going beyond this may be counter productive and lead to frustration and resistance.

> ## Tips
> ### Training sessions - How long?
> According to the master trainers at the famous Spanish Riding School (located in Vienna, Austria), the optimal length of a training session is about 30 minutes (excluding warm-up and cool-down).

Remember that this applies to focused training. This does not apply to pleasure riding, or other activities where the horse is not under strict control and physical pressure. Cherish opportunities to take your horse on a relaxing trail ride where both you and your horse can decompress.

Use repetition

Horses learn best by physical repetition with consistent cues administered with precise timing. When you begin training specific skills, such as backing up, you will find that from day to day, you will have good days and bad days. Over a period of weeks, your horse will improve to the level of his abilities, but do not expect quick learning. It is very important to have patience, and to not become frustrated during periods when your horse seems to forget that which was performed flawlessly the day before!

Horse trainers understand the importance of repetition in horse learning. They also sense when a horse is becoming frustrated, and know when to quit (more about this later). As you develop these skills, it is important to not give up and to use repetition until the activity is ingrained and natural for the horse.

You should expect to take weeks to months or more to train a specific skill to the capability of the horse. It is important to not overdo training on a specific skill after it has been learned. Overdoing training will lead to a bored or resistant horse that will regress into bad behavior.

Use reinforcements

Both positive and negative reinforcements can be used to accelerate the training of your horse. A positive reinforcement may be a rub on the withers, or a tasty horse treat. Your voice can be used to reinforce good behavior with kind words expressed with a calm voice.

Because of the basic pressure/release method of horse training, the majority of horse training activities use a negative reinforcer to ask for the activity (e.g. leg pressure to move forward), followed by a positive reinforcement being the removal of pressure as the horse moves forward.

> ## Note
> ### Horses naturally want to please
> When trained correctly, you will find that your horse works to please you. Herd animals need to "get along" within their herd, so this is natural. If you find yourself frustrated when working with your horse, call it a day.

Uneducated equestrians often look at training techniques and tools as being inappropriate. They frown on the use of spurs, or advanced bits as being cruel or inhumane. The truth of the matter is that tools themselves are not inhumane if used properly by a skilled rider. Indeed, the uneducated use of any bit, or unfailing pressure by a rider is much more inhumane than the use of seemingly advanced tools in the hands of an expert.

The key here is proper education. All serious owners of horses should seek an experienced trainer to help them learn the proper and humane use of tools and aids prior to attempting their use.

Know when to quit

We mentioned earlier the mental capabilities of the horse and how training sessions, especially physically demanding training sessions, should be relatively short. Here we consider not only the horse's capabilities, but also those of the trainer.

When working with your horse, it is critically important to end a training session in a manner that leaves the horse with a pleasant feeling of accomplishment. Never end a training session in abrupt frustration. As you approach the end of your session, ask your horse to do some easy tasks, and provide positive reinforcements through your voice and by rubbing your horse's withers.

Always end your training session with a pleasant cool-down period of walking slowly on a completely loose rein with no leg pressure. Give your horse time to feel good about his accomplishments. You will find that your horse looks forward to training sessions if you always quit the session with some pleasurable activity.

Conclusion

It takes a lifetime of observation and study to learn how horses "think" and why they do what they do. Horses can be charming or nasty - playful or sullen - curious or fearful - social or anti-social - extroverted or intro-verted - indeed the personality of the horse is what make him so much fun to be around.

In this chapter, you learned about the evolution of the horse and why much of horse behavior is based on trying to avoid being eaten. Despite the fact that there are few predators that would tackle an adult horse, that same adult horse may be in absolute panic when a plastic bag blows through its paddock.

You have also learned about the ways the horse perceives the world. How his sight is designed to view to the horizon, both in front and behind. How his sense of smell can detect the slightest scent on the wind of a predator lurking nearby. You have also learned the key to horses and humans working together, the ability of the horse to be desensitized to scary items, to yield to the most subtle pressure, and to work willingly and faithfully.

Horses are excellent communicators, if you know how to listen. This chapter teaches you the basics of horse language. The swish of a tail, the nod of the head, the dancing feet - all are used by the horse to talk to you - to let you know how he feels. If you listen well, you will not only be safer, but your horse will learn faster and enjoy your company.

Lastly, this chapter gives you the tools to learn about how horses learn, and how you can use simple learning theory to accelerate your horse's training and to avoid common problems that resulted from "old-school" training techniques.

Top-5 takeaways

1. Horses act the way they do because of how they evolved. Understanding this basic concept allows you as a horse owner to act in a manner that builds a relationship with the horse.

2. Horses perceive the world differently than humans. They focus on the horizon and are fearful of novel objects. With training, horses can become desensitized to many circumstances, but this training must be compatible with each particular horse's manner of learning.

3. A responsible owner becomes an expert in reading the horse's body language. The ears and eyes are particularly expressive. The wise horse owner learns to read and use body language for safety and communication.

4. When horses are maintained in captivity, environmental factors may lead to stable vices (stereotypies). These behaviors are almost impossible to cure, but in most cases you can prevent stereotypies by addressing the physical and social needs of your horse.

5. Training a horse can easily be accomplished using pressure and release techniques. An understanding of learning theory, and patience are required, along with the physical skill and ability. However, because of the danger involved, basic training is best performed by a professional.

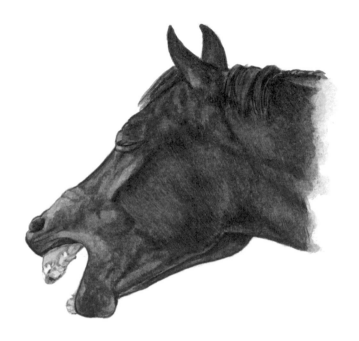

Chapter 2 Dental Care

Introduction

Many new horse owners are surprised when they find that dental care is an important part of horse care. Horses aren't often subject to the types of dental issues that people have. For example, horses seldom get cavities, and in general, have fewer problems with their teeth than we do. However, one major difference between our teeth and horse's is that horse teeth continue to grow throughout their lives. This leads to some unique problems that must be considered by the horse owner.

In this chapter, we will discuss dental care for your horse. You will learn why your horse needs a dentist, and also learn about the diseases and conditions that may result from a lack of dental care.

When putting together your horse healthcare team, you should view the equine dentist as a very important member. Fortunately, most horse oriented veterinarians offer dental care services, so your equine dentist may very well be your equine doctor!

Tooth related conditions are a major cause of premature horse death. A well cared for horse can live 30+ years, and nothing is more rewarding than caring for a been-there done-that senior horse. They are a pleasure to ride and generally fun and safe to be around. Don't shorten your horses comfortable life by ignoring periodic dental care.

Equine teeth

Nature largely took care of the horse's teeth in the wild. Because of the efficiency of the different fibrous textures of the grass, plants, twigs, and tree limbs that horses grazed on, their teeth usually wore down more evenly than those of our domesticated horses. In addition, no bits or bridles took a toll on the wild horse's teeth. The situation for the modern domesticated horse is drastically different from that of the wild horse when it comes to the need for dental care. The domesticated horse's diet is much different. Many horses spend little time foraging for their feed. Instead they are fed softer kinds of hay, commercial feeds, supplements, mashes and other feeds that don't affect their teeth in the same way the forage affected the wild horse's teeth and mouth.

Warning
Avoid a crushing bite

Horses have powerful jaws that can easily crush or sever a misplaced finger. Do not put your hands or fingers in your horse's mouth unless you know how to do it safely. Ask your veterinarian to show you how to examine teeth safely

In addition, the breeding of horses over the years has led to changes in the way some horse's mouths and teeth develop. With out correction by a knowledgeable equine dentist these conditions can make eating difficult, leading to other health problems. As a result, most horse's teeth need floating and dental care on a regular basis to keep their teeth healthy and in proper form. In addition, the use of bits and bridles along with other conditions that affect horses dental health such as periodontal disease, abnormal wear patterns, and broken or cracked teeth make a regular dental checkup as important for a horse as it is for a human. According to veterinarians, taking care of your horse's teeth with routine dental care can add as much as ten years to your horse's life.

Dental changes through your horse's lifetime

When a foal is born, it normally has no teeth, but that changes soon after foaling with the eruption of incisors, cheek teeth and molars. As in all areas of the developing fetus and later the foal, the oral cavity and

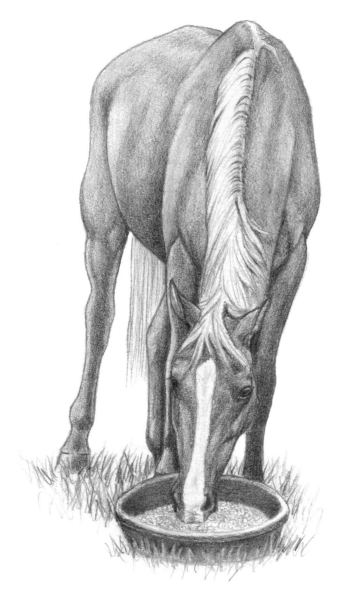

Digestion begins here
Healthy and sound teeth are required to break down the coarse foods that horses consume.

the dental system in the horse develop via a complex series of events that begin at conception. A young foal has 24 deciduous teeth also known as milk or temporary teeth by the time it is approximately nine months old. These deciduous teeth are replaced during the next five years with between 36 and 44 teeth appearing by the time the horse is five years old. The average number of permanent teeth in a male horse is 40, with an average of 36 permanent teeth in a female horse. This variation in number of teeth occurs because a male horse often has several canine teeth, while they are either absent or rudimentary in the mare and some horses have wolf teeth that don't need to be removed.

> ## Note
> ### Quidding
>
> If you observe your horse dribbling wads of hay or grain out of the corners of his mouth, you are observing quidding. This action may indicate that the horse's teeth are not correctly grinding the food and require attention.

The top surface or crown of the horse's tooth is covered by hard enamel which is resistant to bacteria and acids. Underneath the enamel is the dentin which is a softer material. Beneath the dentin is the pulp of the center of the tooth that contains blood vessels and nerves. The root of each tooth is covered by cementum that attaches the tooth to the periodontal membrane which connects to the bony socket in the horse's jaw. The teeth of a horse are much longer than human teeth with up to four inches of tooth imbedded in the bone of the upper and lower jaws. A horse's teeth continue to grow or erupt throughout the horse's lifetime growing at a rate of approximately 1/8 inch each year. They are continually being worn down by the grinding action necessary to thoroughly masticate the feed the horse eats.

Teeth begin the digestive process

Unlike some animals that can digest their food with little breakdown by chewing, horses must chew their food sufficiently for it to digest properly and receive maximum nutrition. If the horse's teeth don't have a flat surface that can grind the food, the digestive process is hindered. In the process of grinding the feed, the horse's jaw moves both up and down and from side to side. Because of the structure of the horse's jaws and teeth, this grinding action often causes uneven wear on the teeth resulting in sharp points that need to be removed or floated on a regular basis so the horse can chew its feed satisfactorily.

A horse's teeth are arranged so that they can properly masticate forage and grain into the bits and pieces that can be processed in the digestive system. At the front of the horse's mouth are the incisors which are used to bite or cut off pieces of feed. Most horses have six incisors on the top and six on the bottom for a total of twelve incisors.

Canine and wolf teeth

A male horse usually has up to four canine teeth in back of the incisors and in front of the three premolars. These teeth are tusk-like and sometimes protrude.

Wolf teeth which are extra teeth are remnants of the first premolars and may be found adjacent to the front premolars. They are often needle-like, and, if they interfere with the bit or cause alignment problems, they should be extracted, usually at 18 to 24 months.

Premolars and molars

Next in position are the premolars, three in number on each side of the upper and lower jaws for a total of twelve premolars.

Behind the premolars are additional molars also known as cheek teeth or jaw teeth. These twelve molars are evenly divided on each side of the upper and lower jaws. The horse's molars do the major work of grinding the horse's feed so it can be digested satisfactorily.

Between the cheek teeth and the incisors or canine teeth of most horses is a space known as the interdental space. This space provides a place where the bit can rest without having the jaws open or having the bit rest uncomfortably on the horse's teeth. In some cases, a veterinarian or equine dentist will file a "bit seat" in the first cheek tooth if the horse does not have adequate natural space in his mouth for the bit to rest comfortably. In all cases the correct bit for the horse should be selected and care should be taken in adjusting the bridle so that the bit does not rest too low or too high, where it pushes against the teeth causing discomfort.

The equine dentist

Equine dentistry was practiced as long ago as 600 BC in China, and has long been important as a method of assessing the age of a horse. Currently, in the United States, some veterinarians go beyond the training required to become a veterinarian by taking additional courses to become

Advanced Certified Equine Dental Practitioners. This advanced training, allows them to effectively promote equine health and balance from head to toe. Using their knowledge of anatomy, physiology, head, mouth and tooth structure, along with their specialized dental skills, they are in a position to diagnose and treat all kinds of equine dental problems whether major or minor.

Many states allow a licensed Doctor of Veterinary Medicine (DVM) to perform all aspects of equine dentistry without any additional certification. As veterinarians, they can use sedation and motorized dental tools in the treatment of equine dental problems, but may not have the knowledge and skills to treat more serious equine dental problems. Most veterinarians continue to take courses not only to stay up-to-date on the latest developments in equine care, but also to learn about advancements in technology and medicine that can be of benefit to their clients.

Some equine dentists get their start by becoming equine dental technicians. To become a dental technician, they must receive focused instruction in a variety of courses including equine anatomy, physiology, tooth structure, and performance dentistry. Dental technicians must work with a licensed veterinarian in dental practices involving sedation and use of motorized dentistry tools. After their initial training, most dental technicians do an apprenticeship with an established equine dentist. Along with practical experience, they usually take frequent classes to up-date and polish their skills.

Equine dentistry has seen growth in effectiveness during the last few years due to technological advances and recognition that proper dental maintenance is essential to prevent premature tooth loss and promote complete utilization of feed. Good dental health helps reduces cases of impaction and gas colic, keeps the horse's mouth in good shape, and promotes peak performance and harmony between the horse and rider.

Skill requirements

Equine dentists spend the majority of their time performing preventive dentistry on horses. Horse's teeth must be floated on a regular basis to smooth the sharp points that develop on the horse's teeth as a result of chewing hay and grain. This is usually done manually with a rasp. If not done on a regular basis the sharp points can cause mouth pain and cuts that not only hurt the horse, but create bit and riding problems. Equine dentists also remove tartar, treat dental caries and periodontal disease,

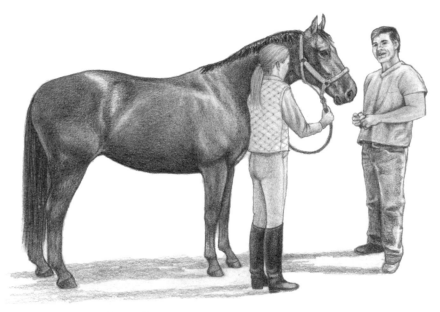

The Equine Dentist

In most cases, your veterinarian will provide dental care for your horse. For special needs horses, you may wish to find a dental care specialist. Ask your veterinarian for assistance.

and, when necessary, extract teeth and remove caps or deciduous teeth.

Effective equine dentistry requires a love and understanding of horses along with compassion and patience. Excellent communication skills are necessary to explain procedures, risks and possible outcomes to owners of horses.

Dental exam

By the horse owner

Learning to check a horse's teeth is an important skill for all horse owners and should be a priority both to save your horse from rapidly developing dental problems, but these exams can also save you both time and money when it comes to good dental care for your horse

If you have not been touching and handling your horse's muzzle and mouth area on a regular basis, have your equine dentist or veterinar-

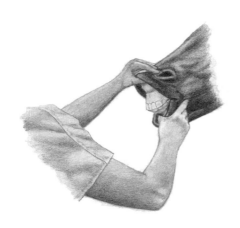

Checking teeth

A limited but useful check can be performed by the owner. You may observe retained caps, broken teeth, or some common malocclusions.

ian show you how to do it safely. Horses have tremendous chewing power and your fingers and hands are at extreme risk when in close proximity to the horse's teeth.

You as a horse owner can take a proactive role in promoting good dental health in your horse by routinely touching and handling your horse's head and mouth area to make the horse comfortable with having the mouth examined. Not only will the horse be more relaxed and comfortable during floatings and dental procedures, but this will enable you to spot any problems early.

By the equine dentist

Only a minimal exam can be done by the horse owner. To adequately examine the horse's teeth, a speculum must be used to allow observation of the molars that are well out of reach for the horse owner. Your equine dentist will fully inspect the mouth and be able to diagnose and treat problems that cannot be observed or diagnosed without proper equipment and skill. If you have handled your horses face and muzzle consistently, and performed superficial examinations of the front teeth and forward molars, your horse can probably be examined by your vet without sedation. This saves you money, and also saves the horse from unnecessary sedation.

Veterinarians generally recommend an annual dental exam. Teeth should only be floated if a problem exists. The length of the teeth are truly finite, and removing the tooth material hastens the day when there is no more tooth to emerge. Because of this, power floating should only be done if necessary!

Dental exam for the foal and young horse

With any new foal, it is important that the foals teeth are examined as soon as possible. Checking for baby teeth called caps that are pushed out by the growing permanent teeth by the time the horse is about two years old is important. If caps are creating pain and soreness in a young horse, you may have your veterinarian remove the caps. The same goes for wolf teeth that are extra teeth and may grow in crooked or in the wrong spot.

Dental exam for the adult or aged horse

With an adult horse, the owner should open the mouth and check for uneven wear on teeth resulting in points or sharp edges that will keep the horse from properly chewing feed on a regular basis. Also note any teeth that are beginning to protrude excessively or cause mal-alignment or malocclusion.

Horse owners need to be aware of any changes in eating habits, loss of weight, bad breath, dropping half-eaten food, holding the head at a strange angle, bolting or head tossing when being bridled or ridden in their horse. These conditions are often caused by dental problems that cause the horse pain or discomfort.

Again, it is money well spent to have either a veterinarian or an equine dentist evaluate the horse's dental health as soon as possible to prevent serious threats to the horse's well being.

Dental speculum

A complete dental exam requires the use of a specialized speculum. Without this device, the rear teeth are impossible to properly examine.

Common equine dental treatments

Floating (abrading)

The most common treatment for equines is the process of floating or rasping the teeth also referred to as equilibration. This procedure should be performed on a routine basis geared to the needs of the horse which may be every 6 months to once every couple of years. The procedure is not painful to the horse and can usually be done with minimal restraint with an assistant holding the horse's head, although excitable horses may need to be tranquilized. Floating corrects minor abnormalities of wear and controls sharp edges and points that develop as the horse chews its feed.

Tartar (cleaning)

Tartar removal is necessary with some horses. This yellowish build-up of organic and inorganic substances that accumulate on the horse's teeth is usually removed with the use of air abrasion, dental picks and other scraping instruments. Individual metabolism or chemical makeup in the horse's mouth will affect how often tartar needs to be removed.

Gums

Periodontal pocket repair helps keep the horse's mouth, teeth, and bone structure in a healthy condition. When periodontal pockets form, the gums separate from the teeth resulting in mechanical and toxic bacterial damage to the tooth. If not corrected, these infected, bacteria-laden pockets may damage the gums and lead to loss of the tooth. The equine dentist will remedy this problem by irrigating and debriding the affected area using compressed nitrogen, water and aluminum oxide powder along with disinfectants. When necessary, a prescription for antibiotics may be necessary.

After a thorough dental exam, the equine dentist will usually follow through with the dental care and work that the examination calls for. In most cases, the equine dentist will go over the problems observed during the examination, give details about treatment and cost of treatment, and answer any questions you, as the horse owner, might have. As your horse gets older, frequency of exams should be increased because of possible periodontal disease caused by a break down in tooth and gum structure leaving food and bacteria trapped in gaps or holes created by loss of teeth, fractured teeth or tissue damage that develops as the horse ages. In such cases, the horse may need corrective work along with a series of antibiotics for the mouth to completely heal.

Dental diseases and conditions

Domestication and breeding of horses through the years has led to dental diseases and conditions that were rare in the wild horse population.

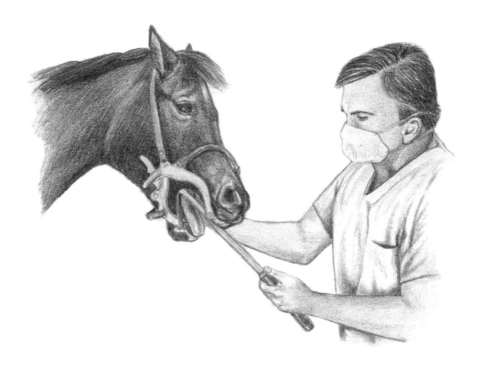

Traditional float

The most common dental operation is called "floating." The equine dentist
uses an angled rasp to remove sharp edges called hooks and points, to assure
that the horse is able to correctly chew his food.

Given the grazing nature of the wild horse, the variety of twigs, grasses,
and tree bark that made up the horse's diet helped to keep the horse's
teeth and mouth relatively healthy. If a wild horse had serious mouth or
teeth defects, the chances of it surviving long enough to affect the gene
pool were rather slim, so serious defects were not passed down to future
horses for the most part. Like modern-day people who often have diets
of processed foods that require little chewing and can lead to cavities,
periodontal disease and other dental problems, domesticated horses also
are subject to a variety of dental problems. A few are inherent or genetic,

others result from the horse's diet, accidents, or disease.

Common equine dental issues

Missing teeth are fairly common in horses. They are usually caused by failure of normal development of a tooth bud. In most cases, the missing tooth is "filled-in" by the teeth on both sides, and the mouth appears normal. If the missing tooth doesn't create a problem with chewing, no treatment is necessary. However, a missing tooth that leaves a gap with an unopposed tooth on the other side will require special attention. See malocclusions below for more about these common dental problem.

Some horses have canine teeth which are large and tusk-like in form. They are commonly found in male horses and may need to be rasped down to prevent interference with the bridle or bit. A canine tooth that fails to erupt may cause a cyst in the gum which should be evaluated by an equine dentist or veterinarian if it causes sensitivity in the gum.

Dental caps in horses are deciduous or temporary ("baby") teeth that remain attached to the permanent teeth after they have erupted. The caps can be extremely sharp and may cut the cheek or tongue and interfere with eating. The caps normally fall off without intervention, but some caps may be retained and should be pulled off by your equine dentist to prevent other dental problems. Dental caps should be removed once the adult teeth have emerged from the gum line.

In some horses, long sharp points may develop on the first upper cheek teeth known as the second premolars and the last lower cheek teeth, the third molars. These sharp hooks can cause a malocclusion problem and the long sharp points may lacerate the gums and make eating painful. Small hooks can be filed off, and large hooks should be cut off. The process of filing down these hooks and points is called "floating".

As in humans, when a horse has a foreshortened upper or lower jaw, insufficient room may exist for the teeth to erupt normally. When the teeth cannot come through, they become impacted. If the impacted teeth become infected or create chewing problems, they need to be extracted. Retained incisors are similar to dental caps except that the retained incisors are in front of the permanent incisors. These incisors should be extracted to insure a correct bite.

Broken teeth

Older horses may develop fractured or cracked teeth. While these teeth may not cause any problems especially if the split doesn't extend below the gum line, they need to be examined periodically to make sure they are not damaging the horse's mouth. If damage to the broken or split tooth involves the root or surrounding bone, the tooth should be removed. The main problem with a split or broken tooth is that the opposing tooth will not be ground down during the eating process resulting in increased length that may interfere with chewing. In this case, the opposing tooth should be floated or rasped frequently to prevent mouth injury.

Many horses have super-numerary teeth which are excess teeth that develop due to the splitting of a tooth bud. These excess teeth create dental crowding that push other teeth out of alignment and may cause gum infection and tooth decay. If the extra teeth injure the gums or cheek, they can be filed or trimmed. In some cases, supernumer-ary teeth should be removed to keep the regular teeth properly aligned.

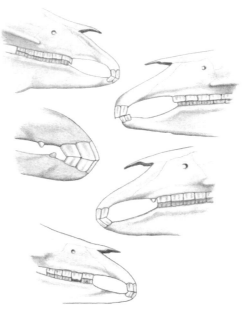

Common dental conditions

These horse skulls exhibit some typical orthodontal problems that are observed in horses. Clockwise from top-left: Wave Mouth, Parrot Mouth (overbite), Wolf tooth, Malocclu-sion due to missing tooth, Canine teeth.

Wolf teeth are often present in the upper jaw of a horse and are vestiges of the first premolars. Delay in eruption and displacement by the second premolars may cause abnormal alignment. If sharp points develop they may lacerate the cheeks and tongue. When this occurs, wolf teeth should be extracted. Wolf teeth can also interfere with the bit, and when this occurs, they should be extracted at 18 to 24 months of age.

Abnormal chewing patterns, along with susceptible teeth that may be softer than other teeth, often result in wear problems that tend to be progressive and become worse with time. Not only do these wear patterns interfere with eating, but they also affect the performance of the horse because of interfering with the bit, causing weight loss and making digestion of feed more difficult.

Three kinds of wear problems in horse teeth
Smooth Mouth

When both the enamel and dentin wear down at the same time, the rough grinding surface of the cheek teeth becomes smooth and the horse cannot grind its feed properly as it chews. Weight loss, digestive ailments such as colic, constipation and malabsorption occur. If the smooth surfaces are the result of improper floating, they may self-correct over a period of time. In other cases, there is no effective treatment and the horse's diet will need to be changed to soft mashes, chopped wet hay, or processed grain.
Step Mouth

Changes in the height of adjacent premolars and molars result in this disorder. A lost tooth or a retained dental cap may cause step mouth which is a serious problem because of the difficulty the affected horse has in chewing and digesting food. Treatment involves cutting elongated molars and rasping the teeth at regular intervals to prevent the step effect.
Wave Mouth

Wave mouth usually occurs in older horses and ponies. The crests and troughs created by the wave pattern allow some teeth to become too long and others opposing them, may be ground down to the gum line causing tooth and gum injuries. Mild cases can be corrected by floating the teeth at frequent intervals. In severe cases, rasping, chiseling, and cutting the molars may be necessary to allow the horse to chew properly.

Periodontal disease in horses

Another problem that often affects horse's mouths and teeth is periodontal disease that occurs when the gums become infected and separate from the teeth. Most commonly, this occurs in the upper cheek teeth, but can occur anywhere in the horse's mouth. Horses do not develop cavities in their teeth. Instead, dental infection begins at the root of the tooth and is usually preceded by gum infection. When the gums are infected, small pockets and crevices along the edges of the gums trap food, the pockets and crevices then become infected. The infection works its way into the pulp cavity leading to root abscesses and bone infection. When the bone recedes because of the infection, the roots become exposed and the stability of the tooth is lost often leading to the loss of the tooth. Often the cheek teeth in the upper jaw become infected. The roots of these teeth are imbedded in the maxillary sinuses. When the roots of these teeth are infected, they cause bacterial sinusitis and a foul-smelling discharge

> ## Note
> ### Dental disease - a painful killer
> A leading cause of premature death in horses is the lack of dental care leading to periodontal disease. According to David Klugh, DVM, up to 60% of horses 13 years and older suffer from severe periodontal disease, which, if untreated, can lead to premature death of the horse.

through the nostril occurs. A fistula or abnormal passage may develop between the oral and nasal cavities, making it necessary to extract the tooth to cure the infection.

Common malocclusions in horses

Some horses are born with a congenital malocclusion between the upper and lower jaws causing incorrect bite problems. These malocclusions may lead to mouth infections, poor chewing patterns and impaired digestion that may compromise growth and development. A malocclusion is an abnormality of the coming together of teeth. In some cases, malocclusions are hereditary. In other cases, the malocclusion may result from an accident, or an abnormal behavior. Horses may also have malocclusions that result from behaviors like cribbing, or result from an accidental breakage of a tooth. Because of the continual growth pattern of equine teeth, the lack of dental care may cause a simple malocclusion to become painful for the horse, or even life threatening.

Here are the most common hereditary malocclusions that are present in some horses:

Parrot Mouth

With this deformity, the lower jaw is shorter than the upper jaw, causing the upper incisors to overhang the lower incisors. The upper incisors become elongated and grow like rabbit teeth. If detected at an early age the problem can be treated by applying wire tension bands to the upper jaw, thereby slowing its rate of growth.

Sow Mouth

Sow mouth is the opposite of parrot mouth with the lower incisors projecting beyond the uppers much like those in a bull dog. This condition is less common than parrot mouth.

Shear Mouth

Shear mouth is related to a widening of the upper arcade of teeth making it much wider than the lower arcade. This produces uneven wear on the teeth with extremely sharp shearing edges developing on the cheek teeth. Older horses often develop this problem with age-related changes involving the shape of the mandible.

Veterinarians often recommend that horses with malocclusions not be used for breeding because most malocclusions have an hereditary basis.

When dental problems with your horse arise, always consult an equine dentist or a veterinarian with special training in equine dentistry.

Dental procedures

With horses now living for twenty to thirty years and older, many horse owners recognize the value of making sure their horse's teeth receive regular checkups and care to catch dental problems before they affect over-all horse health

What to expect from your equine dentist

After a thorough dental exam, the equine dentist will usually follow through with the dental care and work that the examination calls for. In most cases, the equine dentist will go over the problems observed during the examination, give details about treatment and cost of treatment, and answer any questions you, as the horse owner, might have.

The kinds of dental treatment your horse may receive can be broken down into four different categories with the process of floating or rasping the teeth also referred to as equilibration being the most common procedure in most horses.

This procedure is usually performed on a routine basis geared to the needs of the horse which may be every 6 months to once a year. Floating the horse's teeth is not painful to the horse and can usually be done with minimal restraint with an assistant holding the horse's head, although excitable horses may need to be tranquilized. Floating corrects minor abnormalities of wear and controls sharp edges and points that develop as the horse chews its feed.

As with humans, tartar removal is also an important part of good horse dentistry and is necessary with some horses, The yellowish build-up of organic and inorganic substances that accumulate on the horse's teeth is usually removed with the use of air abrasion, dental picks and other scraping instruments. Individual metabolism or chemical makeup in the horse's mouth will affect how often tartar needs to be removed.

Periodontal pocket repair is often necessary and helps keep the horse's mouth, teeth, and bone structure in a healthy condition. As in humans, when periodontal pockets form in the horse's mouth, the gums separate from the teeth resulting in mechanical and toxic bacterial damage to the tooth.

If not corrected, these infected, bacteria-laden pockets may damage the gums and lead to loss of the tooth. The equine dentist will remedy this problem by irrigating and debriding the affected area using compressed nitrogen, water and aluminum oxide powder along with disinfectants. When necessary, a prescription for antibiotics may be necessary.

Although horses usually don't develop cavities like humans do, problems can occur with pits, chips, splits, breaks, and other conditions that compromise the tooth. Bonding agents, epoxies, and restoration techniques are used to correct any damage to the horse's teeth. These repairs prevent tooth loss, fracturing, and cupping problems that affect the horse's ability to chew properly and also prevent problems with bits and bridles during riding and training exercises.

Signs that your horse has dental problems

During daily once-overs, horse owners should consistently check their horse's mouths for any signs of difficulties with the horse's teeth or mouth. Paying attention to the way a horse eats its feed can also be a key to the horse's mouth health. Sure signs that a horse needs a thorough dental checkup include:

- Difficulty in chewing, with food dropping from the mouth
- Excessive salivation
- Undigested grain and food particles in manure
- Loss of weight
- Not wanting to have face or muzzle handled
- Resisting having the bridle put on
- Head tossing and difficult handling when riding
- Facial swelling

- Mouth odor
- Unpleasant nasal discharge

How the equine dentist goes about floating a horse's teeth

Floating the horse's teeth on a regular basis helps prevent the problems related to uneven or problem teeth and the effect they have on the horse's health and vitality.

Equine dentists make use of specialized tools to quickly and painlessly float a horse's teeth.

Typically, the veterinarian or horse dentist may sedate your horse, not to relieve any actual pain since your horse doesn't have any nerves at the surface of the tooth where floating is performed, but to relieve the horse's anxiety and make the process easier and safer.

A special halter is often used with a rope attached to a beam to hold the horse's head up during the procedure. A mouth speculum is inserted to keep the horse's mouth open, and the equine dentist uses a special tool to rasp off excess tooth material and create a level surface so the molars can come together with proper movement of the jaw. The teeth will not be completely flat or smooth because some irregularity is needed for the horse to grind food.

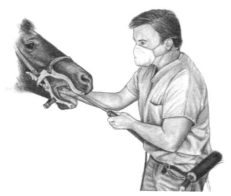

Power float

This dentist is using an electric power float. Power floating provides more control and quicker action, but requires a specially trained veterinarian for proper use.

Once the floating is complete, the veterinarian or dentist will check to make sure the horse's canine teeth are not so long that they press into the opposing gums. If needed, they will be ground down or cut with a dental tool. Some horses have wolf teeth, small premolars on the upper jaw. If present, they will usually be removed.

Horses that have had significant dental misalignment may have a very sore jaw after floating. The horse may have difficulty chewing and grinding food, so appropriate doses of phenylbutazone may be administered and the diet should be supplemented with ground feed until the mouth stabilizes and pain subsides.

Preventing horse dental problems

If your horse's teeth are regularly floated and cared for, most dental problems will be avoided. Depending on your horse's diet, hardness of teeth, and jaw alignment, floating may be necessary on an annual basis, depending on what your veterinarian/dentist prescribes.

Make sure you check your horse's teeth on a regular basis. By noticing any changes in dental surfaces or eating habits, you can be proactive in making sure your horse gets needed dental care. By taking the time and making the effort, you will avoid complications that could affect your horse's health and vitality, as well as the enjoyment you get from your horse.

A Word of Caution: Do not attempt to reach into your horse's mouth and feel the teeth unless you have been taught safe methods for doing so. The horse may bite, or you may shred your fingers on a sharp edge or point of a tooth.

When you as the horse owner or your equine dentist find that a horse has less than excellent dental health, changes can often be made in feeding strategies to promote better dental health

Although older horses most often have dental problems that need special attention, horses of any age may need special feeding strategies because of tooth and mouth irregularities, and digestive problems. Many older horses have difficulty chewing properly, as do some younger horses. Whether it is because of lost teeth, worn teeth, gum problems, or jaws that are misaligned and don't work well together, making chewing and eating easier will result in better nutrition, a healthier horse, and less waste of good feed.

One important point to examine in determining the best feeding strategy for any horse is the form of the feed being given to the horse. Adding some warm water to the feed 10 to 15 minutes before feeding will allow the dentally challenged horse to chew and swallow more easily and will also reduce the chances of choking and colic. This works well with grains and supplemental feeds. In addition, the selection of the feed is important. A senior horse feed with a high fat level of 6 - 10% and containing highly digestible fiber sources, such as beet pulp, is easily digested and can replace much of the hay that the horse would normally consume when a horse is unable to chew regular hay.

Adding some higher quality hay to promote intestinal motility to the horse's feed promotes better absorption of nutrients. Although most senior feeds are high in fiber and can be fed as complete feeds, the horse needs enough bulk to improve intestinal motility. Hay cubes or chopped forage can be soaked and mixed into the feed or fed separately. If the horse is able to eat high quality regular hay, separate the flakes and scatter them in small piles so that the horse walks from one pile to another. This will help the digestive tract and will provide a grazing effect for the horse.

Conclusion

Why should you care about having a horse dentist? After all, feral horses in the wild don't have dental care, and they seem to do OK. In reality, feral horses do suffer from the lack of dental care, and often die directly or are killed by predators because of weakness related to dental diseases and conditions.

In this chapter you have learned that the domesticated horse is actually at a disadvantage relative to his feral counterpart, partly because of his human-supplied diet of hay and grain lacking the natural abrasives that keep tooth growth in check. Lacking periodic dental care, he is likely to develop dental problems, and to share the pain and shortened lifespan of his feral cousins resulting from inadequate dental care.

Top-5 takeaways

1. Dental care is a basic necessity for all horses in captivity. It is a core component of maintaining overall health and wellbeing.
2. Checkups should be performed annually, but floatings or other procedures may not be needed.
3. Traditional and power floating are the most common procedures to compensate for the lack of abrasives in the food of domesticated horses. Avoid over floating that can be a problem with power float tools. Remember, your horse only has so much tooth available during its life.
4. Dental conditions are very painful, and can lead to expensive surgery

or euthanasia if diagnosis and treatment are delayed.

5. The use of a speculum is essential to observe emerging dental problems. Always have a full speculum exam performed.

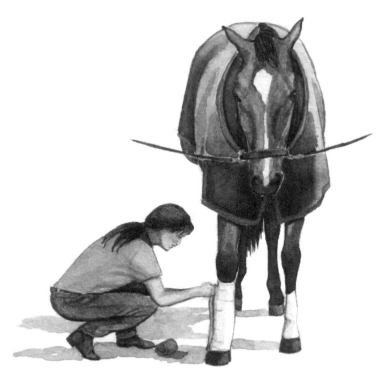

Chapter 3 First Aid

Introduction

The horse evolved living outdoors in the wide open spaces. Horses are diligent observers of their environments and are continuously looking out for predators. "Run first" and "think later" is the typical response of a horse to a perceived danger. As we take our horses from their natural environment, and confine them within barns, paddocks or fenced pastures, we impose barriers that are dangerous to our reactive equines. Beyond the barnyard, your horse also has to cope with trailers, trails and unfamiliar locations that have the potential of causing injury to your horse.

Veterinary care is expensive, and often not available on a moment's notice. Because of this, the horse owner is the first line of care when a minor injury occurs. Learning how to prepare and care for common types of equine injuries will save you money, and also provide quicker relief for your horse. By the end of this chapter you will have a good grasp on the common injuries that you are likely to encounter.

There are classes of injuries that are so serious that early veterinary intervention is critical. You will clearly learn what these types of injuries are so that you won't hesitate to get assistance. You will also learn how to safely handle your horse and how to help your veterinarian by providing handling assistance and diagnostic information, for example how to take vital signs. As you gain your veterinarian's trust, you will be able to handle the level of after care that is required in most instances. While this chapter focuses on first aid, prevention of injury is the goal. You will learn more about prevention in the Healthy Barn chapter.

First aid kit

Having a fully stocked horse first aid kit is vital to proper horse care. It is your responsibility to provide the best care possible for your horses and this means having your first aid kit close by and easily accessible. You can buy a preassembled first aid kit at a tack shop or you can put your own together using supplies you already have and adding others that you purchase at drug stores or wherever you shop.

Remember to check your first aid kit every 6 months and replace any items that are low, missing, dirty or out-of-date. Be sure to include an information sheet with your veterinarian's and farrier's names and phone numbers, address of the nearest equine hospital and phone number, and insurance information if your horse is insured in your kit.

> ## Note
> ### Make vs. Buy
> Pre-made kits are available. These kits contain some basic tools and items, but are generally limited regarding what you will need to have available to handle most situations. In most cases, you can construct a much more useful kit for less money using the list in this section.

The essentials

Here is a handy checklist that you can use to design an excellent first aid kit:

- ❏ Rectal thermometer - digital preferred
- ❏ Water-based lubricant jelly
- ❏ Scissors or knife
- ❏ Anti-bacterial soap
- ❏ Antiseptic wound cleaner such as Betadine® Solution (10% providone-iodine) or Novalsan®

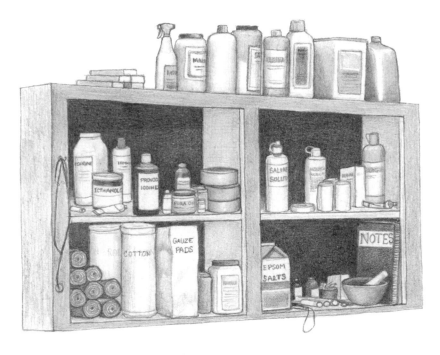

Your Equine Medicine Chest

You will use your well equipped horse medicine chest frequently. It is best to prepare BEFORE the accident occurs.

☐ Surgical scrub such as Betadine® Surgical Scrub (7.5% provi-done-iodine with detergent)
☐ Bandaging material including sterile gauze, cotton, disposable diapers and Tefla® pads, Ace® bandages and self-adherent tape
☐ Leg wraps - both polo wraps and standing wraps
☐ Antiseptic ointment or cream
☐ Furacin dressing
☐ Antibiotic ointment such as Silvadene
☐ Bute for relieving inflammation (prescription medication)
☐ Topical eye ointment and wash
☐ Fly spray
☐ Electrolyte solution or powder
☐ Hoof pick
☐ Tweezers

- ☐ Stethoscope
- ☐ Ice bags or chemical ice pack
- ☐ Epsom salts
- ☐ Zinc oxide cream
- ☐ Clean trash bags
- ☐ Bucket - veterinarians use stainless steel for better sanitation
- ☐ Spray bottle
- ☐ Flashlight with extra batteries
- ☐ Nose or lip twitch for use as restraint

Include any additional medications such as a syringe with tetanus antitoxin and one with tetanus toxoid, oral and injectable antibiotics, tranquilizers, and injectable sedatives and pain killers as recommended by your veterinarian. Also, you should have a small first aid emergency kit for use on the trail, and, if you travel with your horse often, you will most likely want to have a travel first aid kit to be kept in your trailer or truck.

A convenient and portable means of storing your first aid kit is to use a plastic tote bin with lid, available at most home improvement stores. Using a covered tote will keep your kit essentials together, and relatively clean within the barn environment.

When to call the vet

If you have taken to heart the idea that giving your horse a thorough once-over on a daily basis is the smart thing to do is, you are well on the path to being a responsible horse owner.

A daily once-over will save you not only time when a serious illness or injury occurs, but will also save you money spent on veterinarian bills. However, many horse health situations are so important that calling your veterinarian is a "must" because of the dire consequences of not seeking a veterinarian's help in a timely manner.

It's time to call the vet when

1. **Colic symptoms** indicate extreme pain suggesting that the colic is obstructional with possible displacements of parts of the intestine that have become twisted, trapped or pinched in the body cavity, always require a vet's services.

2. **Severe injuries or deep wounds** that expose bone and puncture wounds or wounds that become infected need immediate attention from your veterinarian.

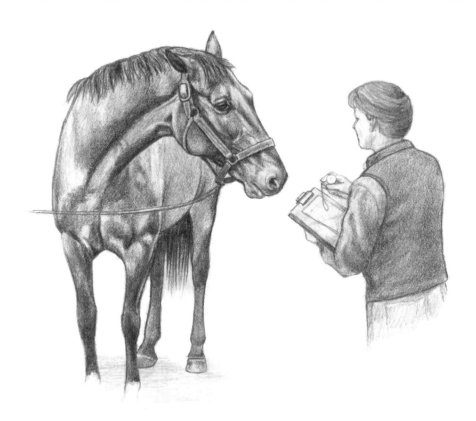

Time to call?

When in doubt, call first and discuss the issue with your veterinarian. Let the veterinarian help you judge the seriousness of the issue and then schedule a visit if needed.

3. **Profuse bleeding** from any part of the horse's body puts the horse at risk for shock and other health consequences.

4. **Inability to stand and lack of coordinated movement** is an indication that the horse has serious health complications resulting from neurological damage or infection.

5. **Severe, watery, foul-smelling diarrhea** can quickly dehydrate your horse and indicates a severe disease or condition that may be life-threatening.

6. **Blood in your horse's urine** indicates a severe infection or bladder injury. Quick, effective treatment is key to minimize damage to

the horse's system.

7. **Choking** on food that has become trapped in the esophagus can lead to damage and scarring of tissue with a subsequent narrowing of the esophagus.

8. **Rapid, labored breathing** or heavy coughing indicate problems that can be life-threatening, and may take diagnostic equipment and a veterinarian's skills to both diagnose and treat the horse.

9. **Eye injury** or condition leading to a painful eye or eyes needs immediate attention by a veterinarian. Corneal ulcers or equine recurrent uveitis which require a vet's attention to prevent blindness.

10. **Swelling** on any part of the horse's body that is hot to the touch indicates infection and needs immediate attention before the infection spreads throughout the horse's body.

11. **Refusal to eat** may simply be is a sign of mild colic, but it can also indicate a severe illness and should be diagnosed immediately.

12. **Straining to urinate or defecate** with nothing or very little coming out may indicate an intestinal or urethral blockage.

> ## Warning
> ### Don't administer pain medicine
> Never administer medicines that may temporarily mask symptoms unless so instructed by your veterinarian. Bute and Banamine and other NSAIDs in particular should only be administered with the awareness and permission of your veterinarian.

It is times like these when it is important to have a pre-existing relationship with your veterinarian. Many veterinarians are reluctant to make ranch visits for new patients and owners in an emergency situation due to liability and safety issues. An emergency visit should never be the first occasion for the veterinarian treating your horse, with the exception of veterinary care at a show, or should you be traveling with your horse.

What to do while waiting for the vet

- **Colic**: Remove all feed and water and calmly walk the horse if possible to relieve discomfort and help pass manure. Monitor vital signs see General Care chapter for how to take vital signs.
- **Choke**: Remove food and water and keep horse calm.
- **Eye injury**: Place horse in a dark stall.
- **Lameness**: If possible move to stall and provide water.

- **Neurological problems**: Place in quiet stall, dim lights and decrease all stimulation possible. Remove all feed.
- **Urinary system**: Check heart rate and collect urine for analysis if possible, especially if discolored, bloody or if horse is straining to urinate
- **Wounds**: Clean and cover if danger of contamination exists.
- **Records**: Check to see when last tetanus booster was administered

Be proactive with prevention

Prevention of situations that create a need to call a veterinarian should always be a priority for horse owners. Before placing your horse in a barn, stable or paddock area, do a simple safety audit to reduce the chances of injury. Use the following check list to help you determine the safety of your horse housing:

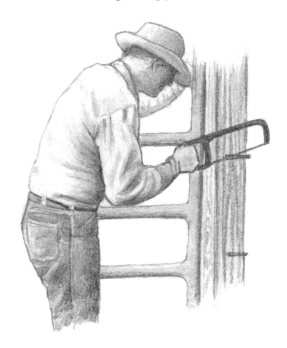

❑ Are pens, gates and fencing in good condition without protruding nails, bolts? Barbed wire should never be used in horse fencing.

❑ Are all gates and doors in good working order?

❑ Are walkways and aisles kept free of debris, and constructed with a rough surface to reduce the chances of slips or falls?

❑ Are wash areas equipped with no-slip

Safe paddocks and barns

The majority of injuries occur in and about the barn due to unsafe conditions. A safety audit is a good idea to remove potential sources of injury.

mats?

❑ Are horse tie posts or rails properly constructed with break-away links or emergency release ties?

❑ Are wires and fixtures protected from contact by the animals?

❑ Are receptacles properly grounded and protected by GFI circuits.

❑ Are baits, poisons, medications and feed concentrates placed in an area inaccessible by the animals?

❑ Are doors and overhead structures sized for horses?

❑ Are paddock areas free of debris, machinery, gopher holes?

❑ Is a fire extinguisher available?

❑ Are horse and human first aid kits available?

You will learn more about barn safety in the Healthy Barn chapter. The point of this safety checklist is to give you a start on reducing the chances of injury by being aware of common problems associated with horse housing.

Handling a sick or injured horse safely

Like any animal that is sick or injured, your horse may respond differently to your attempts to help it. In many cases, the horse will need to be tranquilized or given an intravenous sedative before treatment can begin. The horse's disposition, prior training, amount of pain or fear, the place and extent of an injury, and the duration of the treatment for the illness or injury determines how extensive any restraint will need to be. Often a horse can be calmed by soft talk and a comforting atmosphere.

Danger
Injured horses can be dangerous

A frightened or injured horse can be extremely dangerous and unpredictable. Consider your safety prior to approaching an injured horse, and always take extreme caution to stay out of the flight zone, and be wary of hoofs and teeth that an injured and defensive horse may use.

Restraining your horse

Restraining a sick or injured horse poses one of the most dangerous situations for the horse owner. Extreme care must be taken to remain absolutely calm and to move slowly and deliberately to avoid contributing to the horse's anxiety. In most cases, the halter is all that is needed to restrain the horse for first aid purposes.

Halter and head restraints are used to gain control of a frightened or stubborn horse. Once the horse is calmed and under control, a chain under this chin or across the gums can be added to further control. The head restraint is used for procedures that are relatively minor and painless. An assistant holds the lead and diverts the horse's attention while standing on the same side as the person doing the procedure.

> ## Warning
> ### Veterinarian safety
>
> In most circumstances, when holding your horse for a veterinary procedure, you should position yourself on the same side of the horse as the veterinarian. This will allow you to control your horse's dangerous hindquarters to prevent a kick by pulling the horse's head toward you.

Twitch restraints are considered by some to be similar to acupuncture since they are thought to release endorphins and produce a calming, sedative-like action. Skin, are used most often. A skin twitch is accomplished by grasping a fold of skin in front of the horse's shoulder. This may provide enough distraction for a short procedure. The skin twitch is very useful when giving injections into the neck of the horse.

Hobbles are used to restrain one or more of the horse's legs from movement with a rope-like or strap device called a hobble. Horses need to be trained to accept a hobble, and hobbling should only be done by skilled horsemen to avoid injury to the horse.

Intravenous sedation is used with a horse that resists physical restraint or when a painful procedure is necessary. Phenothiazines such as Acepromazine act on the central nervous system to produce a calming effect or deep drowsiness; Narcotics such as morphine or Demoral are pain killers; Xylazine combines tranquilizing and pain control.

Stocks or a palpation chute are usually used as restraints for rectal and vaginal examinations. Stocks also work well for dental extractions or surgery on a standing horse.

Tail restraints are used when using a halter and lead would be difficult. The tail is grasped and pulled over the back in a circular wheel while encircling the base of the neck with the other arm. Another tail restraint includes tying a rope to the tail and pulling it straight back. The rope is held by an assistant and is not tied to a stationary object. This restraint works well for rectal and vaginal examinations.

Do not attempt any of these restraint methods without proper instruction and practice. Your safety is the top priority.

Common conditions requiring first aid

Here is a helpful guide to common conditions requiring first aid. Regardless of the situation, a call to your veterinarian is in order for most of these conditions:

- Bites and stings - page 70
- Bleeding - page 72
- Choke - page 74
- Colic - page 75
- Diarrhea - page 77
- Eye injuries - page 78
- Fractures - page 80
- Heat stroke - page 81
- Sunburn - page 83
- Poisoning - page 84
- Respiratory distress - page 85
- Shock - page 87
- Sudden onset illness - page 88
- Wounds - page 90

Bites and stings

Horses not only bite each other, but they also suffer bites by other animals including dogs, cats, wild life animals such as skunks, and snakes. In addition, a horse's environment is friendly to many flies, mosquitoes, spiders, bees and other pests which may make the horse miserable and at times threaten the horse's health.

Symptoms

An insect bite or sting often causes a small lump to develop on the horse's skin, which may be painful or itchy. A small hole, or the sting itself, may also be visible. The lump may have an inflamed area around it that may be filled with fluid.

The bee is the only insect that leaves an embedded stinger behind. In cases of a large number of stings, a horse may go into shock as the result of absorbed toxins, and, rarely, anaphylactic shock can occur.

The most common indication of a bite by an animal or a snake is swelling of an area of the horse's body. Closer inspection reveals either bite marks or, in the case of a poisonous snake, two fang marks at the center of the swollen area. Most bites occur to those parts of the horse nearest the ground, such as the legs or the nose while grazing.

Bites by rattlesnakes, moccasins, copperheads and coral snakes cause tissue swelling and pain at the site of the bite. In severe cases when the horse is bitten on the nose, the entire head, including the eyelids and ears, may become swollen leading to nasal obstruction and difficulty in breathing. If you see the symptoms of your horse going into shock, call your veterinarian immediately.

> ### Note
> #### Watch for the bee imposter
> Small bee-like creatures hovering around your horse's legs, chest or muzzle may be stingless, but can also pose a danger to your horse. These are bot flies that deposit eggs on your horse's hair shafts. Bot larvae are a common horse parasite. If you see bot fly eggs, you can remove them with a bot knife or bot block.

Bites of black widow, Missouri brown spiders and tarantulas can cause chills, fever and labored breathing after the initial sharp pain of the sting.

Causes

Unless horses are confined to barns, pastures and stalls that are kept immaculately clean and free of flies, insects, pests and other animals, they will be subject to bites and stings. Horses that are used for trail riding encounter wild animals and both poisonous and non-poisonous snakes.

First aid

If your horse receives a deep bite from another horse or any animal, call your veterinarian as soon as possible. All bites are heavily contaminated puncture wounds and the possibility of rabies should be kept in mind if your horse is bitten by a wild animal.

Washing or flushing bite areas with tap water which has a very low bacterial count and causes less tissue irritation than sterile or distilled water is important in many cases.

In case of a bite by a poisonous snake, restrain the horse and keep it as quiet as possible to prevent further spread of the venom. If the bite is on the leg, apply a tourniquet or constricting bandage such as a strip of cloth several inches above the bite. Be sure to loosen the bandage every hour for five minutes to maintain some blood flow. To check for proper constriction, you should be able to slip a finger beneath the bandage. Apply cold water packs to the site of the bite at 15 minute intervals while waiting for the veterinarian unless directed otherwise. Do not attempt to irrigate or treat the wound before the horse is sedated because of the possibility of upsetting the horse and increasing absorption of venom.

For first aid treatment of stings or insect or spider bites, first identify the creature that stung or bit the horse. Stings of bees, wasps, yellow jackets and ants all cause painful swelling at the site of the sting. If you see a stinger, remove it with tweezers or scrape a credit card across it to separate it from the skin. Once you have identified the type of sting and removed the stinger, make a paste of baking soda and water and apply it to the site of the sting. If the swelling is significant or if the horse reacts as though in pain, ice packs may be used to help relieve swelling and pain.

After use of the baking soda paste and ice packs, application of a calamine lotion or Cortaid will help relieve any itching or skin discomfort.

After care

Your veterinarian may recommend antibiotics to prevent infection and a tetanus shot if your horse hasn't been vaccinated within the past six months. When your horse is bitten by a snake, your veterinarian may recommend antivenin, corticosteroids, antibiotics, and tetanus prophylaxis along with thorough cleansing and care of the snake bite.

Bleeding

Horses are often subject to injuries where bleeding occurs. Depending on the seriousness of the wound and the amount of blood lost, a wise horse owner loses no time in calling the veterinarian and taking steps to minimize bleeding and damage to the horse's body or legs.

Symptoms

A cut, tear, or slice through the skin of the horse usually results in blood loss. Spurting blood indicates that an artery is most likely involved and calls for immediate action to stop the flow. On the other hand, dark blood oozing through the skin indicates that the bleeding is venous and not immediately life-threatening.

Causes

Injuries to a horse's feet and legs, eyelids, face, ear flaps, mouth, lips and tongue, nostrils and other body parts that cause bleeding are usually caused by contact with barbed wire, nails, and sharp edges on fence posts or other stable or barn fixtures.

First aid

In cases of bleeding injuries, the most important considerations are to stop any bleeding, prevent infection, and to repair the injured area to prevent scarring or further injuries to the horse. Treatment will depend on the extent of the injury, where it is located, and how active the horse is. In most cases of injury to a horse, blood loss is minimal and constant pressure for several minutes will allow the blood to clot. However, if blood is gushing or if application of pressure does not stop the bleeding, a veterinarian should be called immediately.

> ## Tip
> ### Use rolled cotton to cleanse wounds
>
> Veterinarians frequently use rolled cotton to cleanse wounds, as it is relatively inexpensive, and easy to use. Fill a bucket with water and add a squirt of Betadine® solution. Tear off small wads of cotton and put them in the solution in the bucket. Grab a piece of saturated cotton, and starting at the top of the wound, squeeze and wipe downward. Throw the piece of cotton away and get another. Do not reuse!

The injured horse should restrained and a pressure bandages may be used to stop bleeding. The wound should be bandaged securely and pressure applied to reduce the blood flow. If blood is squirting, a tourniquet may be necessary. This is often the case with leg injuries. Call a vet immediately and get advice as to whether the tourniquet might cause harm. A tourniquet should be loosened every 15 to 30 minutes for a duration of approximately 5 minutes to allow blood to temporarily flow back into the limb. Once bleeding is controlled, the injured area should be cleansed, usually by rinsing with regular tap water to remove bacteria and any foreign matter or hair around the area should be clipped, and a disinfectant such as Betadine® solution applied along with an appropriate bandage.

If the area is too large to be bandaged, a clean pad made from gauze or other clean fabric should be placed against the wound.

After care

All injured areas should be checked and rebandaged regularly as healing progresses. If a bandage is not necessary, the area should be kept clean and a veterinarian may recommend a first aid product to aid in healing the injured area. Eyelid, ear flap, nostril, and facial injuries require special care with sutures and treatments to minimize scarring and prevent possible distortion of features or actions. If the bleeding occurs in an area where infection could lead to peritonitis or other acute infections, antibiotics and further treatment to reduce possible infection will be an important part of the treatment. If the wound is deep or near a vital structure, surgical repair by a veterinarian will be necessary once the bleeding is under control.

Choke

Choke is caused by a blockage in the esophagus. The esophagus connects the mouth to the stomach. Generally, a choke does not obstruct the wind pipe, but there is a serious danger of the horse aspirating materials into the lungs resulting from the choke.

Symptoms

When an equine acts nervous, coughs, salivates with his head down, backs away from food, arches his neck and swallows repeatedly, or regurgitates with bits of watery food coming out of his nose and mouth, it is possible that an impaction is keeping food or a swallowed object from moving through the esophagus. The horse will act distressed and show no interest in feed or water.

First aid

First step is to remove all food. If possible, carefully clean out the horse's mouth. If you know it is food and can tell where the impaction is, you may try massaging the left side of the neck over the lump to help move it along. Sometimes, walking the horse while allowing it to lower its head will help move the obstruction. If the horse continues to show distress and indications of blockage in the esophagus after the neck has been messaged and the horse has been walked, it is time to call the veterinarian.

If there is any chance that the impaction is caused by a hard or sharp object, such as a piece of wood, or a large carrot that might cause damage to the esophagus, it is best to wait for the veterinarian. Once the veterinarian arrives, the horse may be tranquilized and a stomach tube passed gently through the esophagus to dislodge the obstruction. Medication to help the esophageal muscles relax and function more efficiently may be administered. If the impaction doesn't begin to dissolve and can't be dislodged, the horse may be placed under general anesthesia so that the veterinarian can use a scope to extract the impaction or move it along into the stomach. In a worst case scenario, the veterinarian may need to surgically open the esophagus and remove the impaction.

After care

An examination should be completed to determine if any damage has been done to the esophagus, or if a tumor or stricture is causing a narrowing of the passage. If damage is apparent, the horse's diet may be restricted for several days, with plenty of clean, fresh water prescribed, followed by feeding of a soft diet.

It is important to correct any dental problems the horse has which prevent thorough chewing of feed. Provide small amounts of feed, especially grains, more frequently and, if necessary, moisten the grain. When feeding carrots or similar

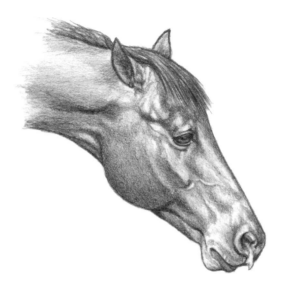

Choke symptoms

Choke is used to describe an obstruction in the esophagus of the horse, and not the air pipe. A horse suffering choke cannot eat or drink, but generally can breathe fine.

foods, make sure they are in smaller pieces that won't cause the horse to choke. If the horse gobbles down food, spread it out or mix it with chopped hay to prevent ingestion in large clumps. When feeding pellets, add a few large stones to the feed box so the horse has to search for smaller bites of feed instead of ingesting large mouth's full.

Colic

Equine colic is not one specific disease, but a symptomatic term. Loosely defined, colic means abdominal pain.

Symptoms

Colic symptoms are generally related to the degree of pain and the horse's ability to tolerate the pain. While some horses will exhibit dramatic signs from even a small degree of gas distension, other horses may be very stoic and show only mild signs in spite of having a severe condition. Generally a colicking horse will move in ways that show it is uncomfortable. It may stretch, paw, get up and down, and roll on the ground. Bloating, sweating, an absence of gut sounds, or turning its head while biting at its sides and flanks may indicate colic. Standing with its head down looking exhausted, loss of appetite, elevated heart and respiratory rates, and trembling are other symptoms of colic.

Causes

Colic in horses can stem from a vast number of causes. Overfeeding, rapid intake of feed, impaction in the digestive tract, parasites, an abrupt change in diet, too much grain, tainted hay, lack of water during lengthy travel, ingestion of sand, and other factors, including stress and long term use of non-steroidal anti-inflammatory drugs such as Bute, are among the causes of colic.

First aid

If you suspect your horse has colic, remove all feed, but make water available in case the horse wants to drink. Let the horse rest if possible and make sure the horse is in a safe area, such as a stall with padding on the floor. Hand walking can be helpful especially for mild cases of gas colic. Do not attempt to walk a horse that is attempting to fling itself to the ground or is rolling about. Always consider human safety first. Do not administer any medication.

Calling your veterinarian at the earliest sign of colic is extremely important since many cases of colic can be treated with medication. More serious cases may require immediate surgery to save the life of the horse. An outwardly calm horse may have a serious problem, while one in apparent agony could have something more mild. Usually the veterinarian will be able to treat the horse on-site. If displacement or impaction is suspected, the horse may be referred to an equine surgical hospital to correct the physical problem.

After care

Caring for your horse after a bout of colic will depend on the kind of colic and the treatment necessary to alleviate it. Obviously, if surgery is necessary, your veterinarian will give you complete instructions about caring for the horse as it recovers. In cases of less severe colic, after care will include taking steps to prevent further bouts of colic. In a case of sand colic, feeding your horse away from sandy ground will help prevent future bouts of colic.

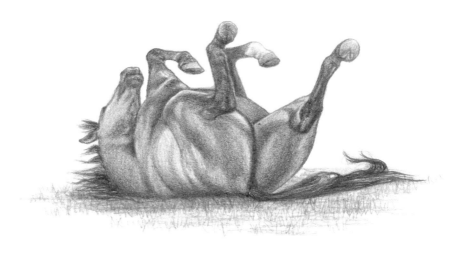

Colic symptoms

Frequent laying down, rolling and a depressed look are characteristic signs of colic. Colic can be deadly, so a veterinarian call is warranted.

Diarrhea

Diarrhea is a condition where a horse expels loose watery manure with an increase in frequency and volume. It is often a symptom of health conditions affecting the horse's internal organs and digestive system.

Symptoms

The loose, watery manure may be dark in color, explosive, foul-smelling, bloody or blood tinged. On going diarrhea causes dehydration and may lead to weight loss, listlessness and obvious discomfort. In foals, unsightly hair loss may occur around the tail area. The horse may have a fever, evidence abdominal pain and abdominal distention may be present.

Causes

Diarrhea can develop as a result of a number of factors, including eating contaminated or unfamiliar feed, overeating grain, ingesting sand or dirt, infection by bacteria or viruses, diseases of the colon, poisoning from plants, arsenic or phosphorus poisoning, parasites, and Potomac horse fever. Shipping or transporting the horse, changing the deworming routine, or treatment with certain antibiotics can also cause diarrhea. Diarrhea is often a symptom of a disease. In cases of chronic diarrhea, it may be caused by diseases of the intestine, such as cancer, or by deficiencies in the intestinal tract that make it impossible for the horse to absorb nutrients. Antibiotics and nonsteroidal anti-inflammatory drugs used over an extended period of time can produce severe diarrhea. In addition, lead and selenium toxicity, plant, and blister beetle poisoning can cause diarrhea.

First aid

First aid treatment includes removal of feed, while providing the horse with plenty of fresh, clean water. Also, a horse with diarrhea should be kept away from other animals.

Any time a horse develops a case of persistent, foul-smelling, watery diarrhea, a veterinarian should be contacted. Be prepared to provide the horse's vital signs, along with information about the loose stool and the state of the horse. Diarrhea can rapidly cause severe dehydration, which can bring on other problems. Initially, the veterinarian will recommend that the horse may need a large volume of intravenous fluid including electrolytes to maintain hydration. The veterinarian may recommend activated charcoal to coat the intestine and decrease absorption of gastrointestinal bacteria through the gut wall. This will give the veterinarian time to diagnose the cause of the diarrhea fully.

After care

Once the horse has been stabilized with rehydrating fluids and electrolytes, the treatment of acute diarrhea is usually directed at the cause. Depending on the horse's condition, antibiotics and anti-inflammatory drugs may be prescribed.

Involving a veterinarian early on, is important in cases of severe diarrhea because secondary complications such as colic, laminitis, and endotoxemia can develop. If the horse's gut has been damaged in any way, the horse may become septic as a result of absorption of gastrointestinal bacteria through the gut wall.

Eye injuries

Injuries to a horse's eyes tend to be traumatic because of the vigorous manner in which horses perform everyday actions. Blows to the eye may cause detachment of the retina, lacerations of the cornea, penetration injuries, and wounds around the eye. Traumatic injuries to horse's eyes range from superficial abrasions to severe lacerations that affect the eye structure. Eyelid abrasions and lacerations are usually obvious and superficial damage may be given first aid treatment. Deeper lacerations that cause squinting, tearing, discharge of mucous or blood require immediate attention from a veterinarian and it is recommended that horses receive tetanus prophylaxis and topical and systemic antibiotics to prevent infection in addition to prompt repair of the damaged eye.

Symptoms

Symptoms of eye injuries include blinking, tearing, or keeping the eye closed because of irritants in the environment or a small foreign bodies in the eye.

Causes

Most traumatic eye injuries are caused by brushing against or running into tree branches or bushes, bumping into fences, banging against stall doors or other objects. The horse's environment inside the barn, out in the pasture, and on trails includes a number of irritants and microscopic particles that irritate or embed themselves in the horse's eyes.

> ## Note
> ### Eye lacerations are always an emergency
> Eye lacerations always require immediate veterinary attention. The eye is very susceptible to infection or irreversible damage if not treated soon after the injury occurs.

First aid

If a foreign body is present, it should be gently removed using a sterile saline flush. Foreign objects such as dust, sand, or plant material that becomes lodged under the horse's eyelids may be flushed with water or saline solution, but any foreign object that pierces the eye ball should not be removed and needs the immediate attention of a veterinarian since microsurgery may be required to remove the object without damaging the eye further.

If the eye appears irritated and there is no sign of injury, it should be monitored closely. If the condition worsens or doesn't improve within 24 hours, an examination by a veterinarian should be arranged. The horse should be placed in a dark environment and kept calm. Small eyelid abrasions and lacerations may be given first aid treatment by cleansing and disinfecting the area. The veterinarian will be able to apply topical anesthetics, and perhaps injectable sedatives so that the horse will allow a thorough examination of the eye.

After care

After care involves watching the horse closely to ensure that the eye is no longer irritated and that it is healing properly with topical treatments if necessary. . Deeper lacerations that cause squinting, tearing, discharge of mucous or blood require immediate attention from a veterinarian and it is recommended that horses receive tetanus prophylaxis and topical and systemic antibiotics to prevent infection in addition to prompt repair of the damaged eye structure by a veterinarian, or in serious cases, an equine ophthalmologist. In some cases, prompt surgical treatment may be necessary.

Fractures

Some horses go their entire lives without breaking any bones, but it is extremely important for a horse owner to know how to provide first aid to a horse that has a fractured bone because, in some cases, the horse's life may depend on proper immediate first aid. Identifying a fracture is not always easy because some fractures are not readily visible such as those in the horse's foot or in smaller bones where no exterior symptoms can be seen.

Symptoms

Bone fractures are classified as open or closed. A closed fracture does not break through the skin. With an open or compound fracture, the bone makes contact with the outside either because a wound exposes it or the broken bone pierces the skin. Open fractures are considered "dirty" because they become contaminated with dirt, debris, and bacteria. Catastrophic fractures are obvious, but horses sometimes fracture a limb in such a way that no break is evident. Instead the horse may appear to be lame.

Causes

High rates of speed and the forces exerted on a horse's leg can lead to fractures. Stepping in a gopher hole or slipping on uneven terrain may cause a fracture. In other cases, a horse may catch its leg in a fence or bump against a solid object with such force that the bone is broken. Bone fractures can occur any time, any place including on the race track, the trail or in the stall or pasture.

First aid

When a fracture occurs, stabilization, pain control, and fracture immobilization are crucial for a positive outcome. Many factors enter into first aid treatment of broken or fractured bones including the site of the break or fracture, whether or not it is involved in direct weight bearing, the age of the horse, and the resources available for treatment. Complete-fracture first aid requires prompt stabilization to reduce the horse's anxiety, thus avoiding further damage. Stabilizing or splinting the fractured limb reduces the horse's anxiety, because it allows him to regain control of the leg even though he can't put any weight on it.

Once the limb is stabilized, most horses will rest the leg rather than try to use it for support. Whenever possible, a veterinarian should apply a splint to a horse's fractured leg. The veterinarian will generally stabilize the leg even before taking x-rays or performing any other diagnostic procedures. In some cases it might be necessary for the veterinarian to sedate the horse to relax him for sufficient splinting. If the horse must be transported to a veterinarian hospital, measures must be taken to minimize movement and keep the horse steady in the trailer.

After care

Infections and destruction of soft tissue can pose problems in the healing process of a fracture. Owners have to be prepared to check casts, change bandages, and take the horse's temperature daily, and evaluate gradual progress to ensure a successful outcome. Once the fracture is healed, the horse may need gradual rehabilitative exercise and a gradual return to normal activity.

Heat stroke

Heat stroke is brought on by a combination of too much exercise and hot, humid weather. Overweight or unfit horses are especially affected.

Symptoms

Profuse sweating, rapid breathing and an increased heart rate are usually the first symptoms. The skin will become hot and dry to the touch while losing elasticity. The horse will cease to urinate and the eyes will take on a dull expression. The horse's rectal temperature may approach 104 degrees or go higher. If heat stroke is not recognized and treated promptly collapse and convulsions may occur.

Causes

A combination of too much exercise and hot, humid weather are the common causes of heat stroke. Heat production can increase as much as 50% during intense exercise. The horse's system may be unable to keep up with the mounting heat to the point that it becomes dehydrated. Horses that are affected by anhydrosis (absence of sweating) are extremely susceptible to heat stroke, and special care should be taken with them since the most important mechanism for heat dissipation in horses is evaporation through sweat. In addition, horses that are unfit or overweight are more

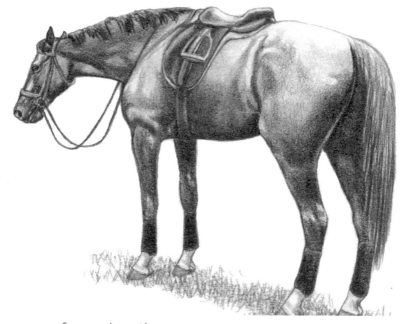

Beware of over-heating

Hot and humid weather can be deadly to your unconditioned or conditioned horse. Take care to avoid heat stroke by being aware of the symptoms and treatments.

susceptible to heat stroke and exhaustion than more fit and lean horses.

First Aid

Immediately move the horse to a cool, shady area and call your veterinarian. Spray or apply cool water to the horse's legs and body, or drape towels soaked in cool water over the horse and around the legs, especially in areas that exhibit large veins. In a critical situation, ice packs may be placed on the horse's legs. Use fans to circulate air if available, and allow the horse to drink small amounts of cool water at frequent intervals, but do not allow drinking of a large quantity of water. Walking the horse slowly in a shady area will help evaporate the heat from the horse's body.

After care

Once a horse has a severe case of heat stroke it may be more susceptible to heat stroke in the future. After a heat stroke, the horse should be watched and gradually returned to the regular exercise routine and workload during cooler times of the day. Knowing your horse's normal vital signs is invaluable in recognizing the seriousness of any case of heat stroke and can serve as a guide to prevent over-exercising the horse when the weather is hot and humid.

Sunburn

Prevention is the best policy when it comes to equine sunburn, but there will be times when your horse will need first aid to reduce inflammation and pain and help the sunburned areas to recover properly before they become infected. Although all horses are susceptible to sunburn, those with light skin, lips, ears and coats are especially susceptible.

Symptoms

In cases of sunburn, the horse's skin reddens, becomes inflamed and painful to the touch. Blisters may form, and the skin may begin to peel. The horse will have symptoms of colic such as pacing, circling and pawing. The horse's appetite will decrease and if not treated promptly, the horse may become sluggish, have diarrhea and lose weight. The horse may develop jaundice.

Causes

Spending too much time in the sun without protective coverings or sunblock will cause a horse to sunburn. In addition, horses on some medications, such as tetracyclines, or with certain diseases, become photosensitive and are more likely to suffer from sunburn.

> ## Caution
> ## Skin cancer concern
>
> Some breeds of horses (Clydesdales, Overo paints and Appaloosas) are suspectable to cancers caused by over-exposure to the sun. Fortunately, sun-blocking lotions and even fly spray can be used to reduce the chances of sunburn.

First aid

Move the horse to a quiet shady area or into a barn or stall and provide plenty of water for the horse to drink to prevent dehydration. If the sunburn is severe, check with your veterinarian as to the best course of treatment. If the sunburn is mild, several good options for treatment are available: Apply a soothing coat of vitamin E diluted with mineral oil over the sunburn area. Apple cider vinegar is also a useful treatment for sunburn in horses. Apply the apple cider vinegar to the affected area several times a day as necessary for healing to take place. Commercial sunburn ointments for children and adults may also be applied to sunburned areas of the horse.

After care

Observe the horse carefully during recuperation to make sure that the sunburn has not affected the over-all health of the horse. The correlation between sunburn and liver damage makes it important to check with a veterinarian in cases of severe sunburn. Prevent sunburn by using a long fly mask, sunblock products or shampoos and conditioners that provide sunburn protection.

Poisoning

Horses often ingest poisons in the form of animal baits, insecticides, toxic plants or forage, improperly stored grain and hay, drugs and medications given in an overdose or by an improper route, household or barn and stable cleaning compounds, paint, and other toxic substances. Since horses are unable to vomit, a plan of action should be in place in case a horse ingests a toxic substance. In any case of suspected poisoning, call your veterinarian at once. If possible identify the source of the poisoning and the type of poison involved. Specific antidotes are available for some poisons. If the poison is known, call the National Animal Poison Control Center at (888) 426-4435. The center is open 24 hours a day. A small charge is made for their services, but is well worth it considering the health of your horse. You may also call your local hospital and ask for information from the Poison Control Center.

Symptoms

Symptoms may vary depending on the type of poison, but in most cases they will include a change in behavior with a lack of ability to perform. Erratic behaviors along with tremors, and a lack of coordination may lead to aimless wandering or staggering, along with difficulty in drinking and eating. Other physical symptoms include a slowed heart rate which may lead to cardiac failure, excessive salivation, discoloration of mucous membranes and difficulty breathing. The horse may lose the ability to urinate, develop symptoms similar to colic and show signs of depression. If untreated, sleepiness, convulsions and collapse may occur.

Causes

The potential list of poisons that may affect horses is long and includes trees, plants, chemicals, medications and drugs, household and stable supplies, venomous snake and insect bites. Ingestion of poisonous plants or forage, contaminated roughage, and improperly stored grain and hay are the most common causes of poisoning of horses. Overdoses of drugs and medications can be deadly, and some horses have allergies that cause them to suffer anaphylactic shock when given a drug by injection.

First Aid

Call your veterinarian immediately if poisoning is suspected. Locate the source of the poison and make sure the horse or other animals do not have further access to the poisonous substance.

Treatment will depend on the type and amount and type of poison ingested or contacted. If the horse has a poisonous substance on its skin or coat, the substance should be washed off with soap and a large amount of water. Mineral or vegetable oil may be used to remove oil, gasoline, or similar products. The oil should be followed by washing with water and a mild detergent.

> # Warning
> ## Be safe - check your pasture
> Before turning your horse loose in a new pasture, take some time to walk around and inspect for toxic plants, gopher holes, and hidden junk. Injury prevention takes a little time, but will save you and your horse in the long run.

Treatment often consists of passing a gastric tube into the horse's stomach to suction and remove the contents. A charcoal slurry may also be administered to neutralize some types of poison. The charcoal slurry is often followed by administration of a laxative to assist the removal of toxic materials from the digestive tract.

Large volumes of intravenous fluids may be required in severe cases, to support circulation, treat shock, and protect the kidneys.

After care

Generally, your veterinarian will advise you about your horse's condition and the prognosis for recovery once the horse has received first aid and veterinary treatment and is on the way to recovery from the poison. Depending on the condition of the horse, it may take some time for the horse to return to a regular, active schedule. Careful observation of the horse is necessary to make sure that the effects of the poison are out of the horse's system before expecting the horse to return to full activity.

Respiratory distress

Respiratory distress in the horse is a symptom of an underlying disease or injury of the lungs. When a horse is in a state of respiratory distress, the emergency requires rapid diagnosis of the problem, a quick assessment as to what will relieve the distress, and procedures to limit any permanent damage to the horse's respiratory system.

Symptoms

Symptoms usually include a runny nose, runny eyes or eye inflammation, coughing, rapid, shallow, or labored or breathing, unusual sounds of breathing such as roaring or wheezing, changes in breathing pattern, (the normal respiratory rate is 6 to 8 breaths per minute) and loss of appetite combined with a fever. If the disease or condition is not addressed, the horse will lose weight, become depressed, lack energy and generally fail to perform.

Causes

The underlying causes of respiratory distress may range from an allergic reaction to dust, mites, or mold spores, to equine asthma to chronic obstructive pulmonary disease or a number of other diseases that cause respiratory distress. Respiratory infections may have viral, bacterial, fungal, or parasitic causes. Upper airway coughs may be caused by respiratory infections, sinusitis, pharyngitis, or guttural pouch infections.

Lower airway coughs indicate acute bronchitis, pneumonia, or possibly the presence of lungworms or the larvae of ascarids. Horses may resort to shallow breathing to avoid the pain of taking a deep breath due to rib fractures, pleurisy, or fluid in the chest. Rapid or labored breathing, which is known as dyspnea, may be the result of fever, shock, dehydration, pain, or fear. Underlying causes include sepsis, heart failure, pneumonia, fluid in the lungs, and chronic obstructive pulmonary disease.

> ## Note
> ### Barn ventilation
>
> A stuffy, dusty barn is likely to cause watery eyes and skin allergies. Keep your horse outdoors as much as possible. Improve barn ventilation by opening doors and windows, even in cold conditions.

First aid

In any case, respiratory distress should be treated as an emergency and consultation with a veterinarian is very important. Calm the horse as much as possible to reduce stress and anxiety. A horse in respiratory distress should be separated from other horses to prevent the spread of any disease, and kept quiet. The stall should be clean, dry, dust-free and well ventilated. If weather is cold apply a horse blanket.

Bronchodilators and a mask inhaler system may be recommended by a veterinarian. Corticosteroids are effective in reducing the inflammatory response brought on by the allergens. If the respiratory distress is a symptom of a disease or condition, appropriate treatment by a veterinarian will be necessary. Vaccines are available for many of the diseases that cause respiratory distress including strangles, rhinopneumonitis, and influenza, although none of them are 100% effective.

After care

A plan to reduce exposure to elements that may trigger respiratory distress needs to be put in place. Good nutrition and stall rest in a well-ventilated setting until the horse has fully recuperated will allow a return to normal routines when the horse is fully recovered. Gradually build back up to your previous work schedule.

Shock

Just as humans go into shock when the circulatory system fails to meet the body's need for oxygen, equines, too, can go into shock.

Symptoms

Typically, an equine that is in a state of shock will appear anxious or agitated, have low or no urine output, may have diarrhea, have a rapid, but weak pulse accompanied by shallow breathing, will sweat profusely and show signs of confusion. As the vital organs shut down because of lack of oxygen, the horse may lose consciousness and without immediate treatment may die. In cases of anaphylactic shock, a systemic reaction occurs and may be accompanied by anxiety, sweating, marked difficulty in breathing, diarrhea, a drop in blood pressure leading to collapse and eventually death, if not treated promptly.

Causes

Common causes of shock are dehydration, profuse diarrhea, excessive sweating, severe colic, heat stroke, snake bite, multiple bee stings, poisoning or major trauma. This life-threatening condition occurs when the body does not get sufficient blood flow to provide necessary oxygen to the brain and major organs. As in humans, anaphylactic shock is caused by a severe allergic reaction to an allergen to which the horse is super sensitive. Multiple bee stings, penicillin antibiotics, vaccines and immune serums are common causes of anaphylactic shock in horses.

First aid

If your horse goes into shock, call your veterinarian immediately. If the horse is unconscious, check and make sure the airway is open, clear secretions from the mouth and pull the tongue forward to prevent blockage of the airway and, if possible, keep the head level with the body.

If the horse is conscious, calm the horse by speaking soothingly and allow the horse to assume the most comfortable position possible to sustain breathing. Control any bleeding from wounds or injuries. If bones are broken, splint or support them before attempting to move or treat the horse. Cover the horse loosely with a coat or blanket.

In severe cases of anaphylactic shock, first aid usually includes administration of epinephrine and possibly glucocorticoids, large volumes of balanced liquids and administration of oxygen. If you know that you have a horse that is susceptible to anaphylactic shock, ask your veterinarian to supply you with a drug such as epinephrine used for emergency treatment. Have your veterinarian teach you how to use it effectively in case of an emergency.

After care

Once the horse is stabilized, your veterinarian will determine the root cause for the shock. In most cases, the cause will be apparent from veterinarian observation and tests, but in cases of severe infection, damage to the nervous system, or foal septicemia, further evaluation and sustained treatment may be needed. A horse recovering from shock will likely be weak and will need careful attention to feeding and access to clean water at all times. Stall rest in a quiet, well-ventilated area is often recommended with a return to normal workload only when the horse completely recovers.

Sudden onset illness

A sudden onset illness is one where the symptoms appear suddenly and seemingly out of the blue. The horse is healthy one minute, but obviously ill the next minute.

Symptoms

Typical symptoms of sudden onset illness include fever, chills, lymph node swelling, nasal discharge, diarrhea and loss of appetite. Other symptoms signaling that all is not well with your horse are depression, stiffness, a change in gait, and loss of coordination. In some cases, paralysis, convulsions and coma may occur depending on the illness.

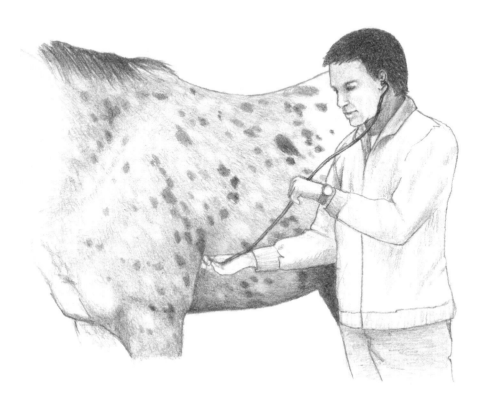

Treating shock

Insufficient blood flow to meet the needs of the horse's organs results in a condition known as shock.

Causes

Diseases caused by viruses, colic, poisonings, adverse drug reactions, hemorrhages, and heart arrhythmias are typical conditions that can appear without warning and need immediate attention.

First aid

If your horse acts unwell and doesn't meet you with the usual vigor that the horse typically exhibits, your first step is to place him in a comfortable, well ventilated area or stall away from other horses. Check the horse's vital signs and compare them with your record of normal readings. Check the horse's mucous membranes for color and also listen for normal gut sounds. Remove feed, but generally having water available is okay unless the horse is choking or coughing. Cool the horse if it has an elevated temperature by sponging it with cool water or spraying gently with a hose. If your horse appears to have colic, you may want to walk your horse to see if that relieves the symptoms. Let your horse choose the physical position that is most comfortable for the horse. If your horse is struggling to stay up, let it lie down. If the horse is down, don't try to get it up. This will only add to the stress of the situation.

Often the veterinarian will be able to make suggestions as to what the causes of the sudden onset illness might be based on knowledge of the illnesses and diseases found in other horses in your area. If the symptoms indicate an emergency that needs immediate veterinarian attention, arrangements for that care and treatment can be made.

After care

The stall or area where the horse is kept should be dry and well-ventilated. If the weather is cold, provide a warm horse blanket, along with clean water and a palatable diet. Exercise should be curtailed until the horse is well on the way to recovery from the illness.

Wounds

Horse wounds generally break down into three types: abrasions, lacerations, and puncture wounds. First aid treatment differs slightly for each type of wound.

Symptoms

An abrasion is a damaged patch of torn skin and hair, which may seep blood and body fluids. As the wound progresses, inflammation occurs and the injured area becomes warm to the touch. Abrasions often have imbedded particles of dirt, grass, splinters, or other foreign matter in them. A laceration is a cut, tear, or slice through the skin of the horse or through the outer covering or membrane of an organ. Depending on the site of the laceration bleeding may be profuse and the wound will begin to swell. Symptoms of a puncture wound include lameness, an uneven gait, a protruding object such as a nail or wood splinter, a gaping hole, a hole that is closed over but bears evidence of a wound, ragged or torn skin and tissue, and sometimes, bleeding.

Causes

Abrasions are usually caused by a horse rubbing against a fence, stall, or other stationary object. Abrasions may also be caused when a horse falls and skids, skinning a hip, leg, shoulder, or other body part. Ill-fitting saddles or saddle blankets that rub repeatedly on the skin, or ropes that are used roughly and inappropriately, may also cause abrasions.

Lacerations to the eyelids, face, ear flaps, mouth, lips and tongue, nostrils, coronet, and feet and legs are usually caused by contact with barbed wire, nails, and sharp edges on fence posts or other stable or barn fixtures They are also caused by neglected teeth, rough handling with tack or bits, contact with hooves or teeth of other horses. Lacerations to the perineum, rectum, vagina, and cervix are usually the result of foal delivery problems, breeding problems, or mishaps during an examination, especially in the case of rectal lacerations.

Puncture wounds are usually the result of stepping on nails, glass, or other sharp objects, although puncture wounds may affect other parts of the horse's body because of falls, accidents, or from collisions with sharp objects.

First aid

In a cases of an abrasion or a laceration, first check to make sure there are no punctures, broken bones, or more serious damage before treating the skin damage. Stop any bleeding by applying pressure with a clean, sterile bandage. If a laceration is bleeding profusely, near an eye or joint, or deep enough that tendons, bone, or internal organs are exposed, a veterinarian should be called immediately. Extensive lacerations

> ## Warning
> ### Puncture wounds - call the vet
> Most cuts, scrapes and bruises can be easily treated by the horse owner. Puncture wounds are another matter. Always call your veterinarian for puncture wounds as antibiotics, even tetanus antitoxin, may be called for.

usually need stitches to heal properly. Small lacerations may not need to be sutured, but care must be taken to make sure they do not become infected and that they are healing properly.

Clean the wound with an iodine-based solution or flush with saline solution to remove dirt, grass, or other particles. If the wound does not look deep, use large volumes of water. Rinse the area repeatedly with diluted Betadine or a similar solution to help clean the area.

Do not rub or scrub these areas as they are tender and you will probably intensify the wound damage. Keep the area moist by using a recommended ointment. Be gentle with the skin area to avoid causing further pain to the horse or more damage to the skin.

Your veterinarian may recommend using Bute to help with the swelling and inflammation. Cover with non-stick gauze and an elastic bandage. In some cases, restricting movement may be helpful while the abrasion or laceration is healing. If the laceration is in a place where infection could lead to peritonitis or other acute infections, antibiotics and further treatment to reduce possible infection will be an important part of the treatment.

Eyelid, ear flap, nostril, and facial wounds require special care with sutures and treatments to minimize scarring and prevent possible distortion of features or actions.

In case of a puncture wound, depending on the origin, depth, size, and location and whether or not the wound is bleeding, a puncture wound should be treated immediately and a veterinarian consulted. Puncture wounds to an area of a horse's body where the internal organs might be affected are extremely serious because of the potential for internal bleeding, infection, and compromise of affected organs.

If the wound is pulsing, that is a sign of arterial injury and you will need to stop the bleeding. You have about 10 minutes before it becomes critical. If you see a penetrating object such as a nail, stop the blood flow as much as possible and leave the object alone until a veterinarian sees the injury. Pulling it out may actually cause more damage.

After care

If the horse has not been immunized against tetanus, prompt tetanus prophylaxis is necessary. To insure proper healing, carefully manage the horse's environment to avoid contamination of the wound by bacteria or other infectious agents that may cause further infection and inflammation.

After care for a puncture wound includes keeping the horse in a clean stall and following the veterinarian's directions regarding further monitoring and treatment. Swabbing the area daily with a 7 percent iodine solution is often advised. Any scabs that form on the surface of a puncture wound should be removed so the wound can heal from the inside out. Vets nearly always advise a course of antibiotics following treatment of a puncture wound to prevent any deep-seated infection.

Conclusion

Horses tend to be accident prone in a barnyard or pasture setting. The general nature of the horse is to react now, and suffer the consequences. Because of this flighty nature, horses are frequently involved in minor to major accidents that result in scrapes, cuts, bruises and all sort of muscle and tendon strains. Preparing for the certain need of first-aid supplies requires a stocked first aid kit.

Using the checklist provided in this chapter, you can stock a barn and trail first aid kit with items that will be used time after time.

This chapter also gave you a basic understanding of horse injuries that you should be prepared for. For each of these injuries, diagnosis, first aid and after care are detailed. This chapter also offers important advice regarding when to call the veterinarian. In some cases, waiting to see if the problem will self-resolve can be dangerous to the health of your horse. It is very important to know when to call the veterinarian. If you have any doubt at all about the care required for any sort of injury or condition, always contact your veterinarian for advice.

Top-5 takeaways

1. Assemble a first-aid kit with commonly used components. You will be surprised how often you use your first aid kit.
2. Get to know your veterinarian before an emergency occurs. Learn when to call the veterinarian. When in doubt, call!
3. Perform a safety audit of your barn, stable or paddock areas. Remove potential sources of injury.
4. Be ready in case of emergency. Learn how to restrain an injured horse, work with the veterinarian safely, and be prepared to transport your sick animal to a veterinary hospital.
5. Familiarize yourself with treatments for common injuries. If you trail ride away from your barn, it is wise to bring along a trail first aid kit.

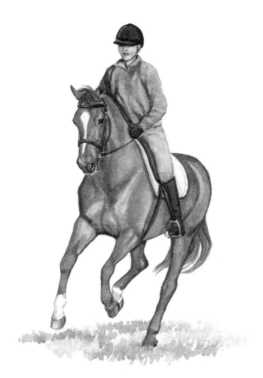

Chapter 4 Fitness

Introduction

One reason many people own horses is to experience nature on horse-back. This pleasurable activity creates a special bond between the trail rider and horse. After hours exploring the local trails, most of us complain about muscle soreness, and fatigue. If only your horse could speak, he would note the same.

Other people enjoy participating in competitive events with their horse, and soon realize the demands made on both the horse and rider when it comes to preparing the horse for competition. When professional trainers are preparing a horse for competition, the first task is to increase the fitness and condition of the horse to where he can be properly trained. Most trainers will ride a competition horse for one hour a day, five days a week.

An hour a day five days a week is more than most "ordinary" horse owners can manage, so there will always be a difficulty in keeping the horse's fitness at a competition level. You can quite easily, however, get your horse to a level of fitness and endurance where he can comfortably be your trail companion or light competitor. To do this, you will need to integrate fitness and conditioning training sessions into part of every ride.

This chapter offers a basic foundation of how to obtain and maintain a level of fitness that will contribute to your horse's mental and physical wellbeing. You will learn how to properly structure your riding sessions to reduce injury, and condition for the type of activity you enjoy with your horse. But, before getting into the development of a fitness training program, let's begin with a foundation based on equine physiology.

> ## Note
> ### Benefits to the rider/trainer
>
> Riding and working with horses is marvelous exercise for humans too. You will notice an increase in strength and balance, and also build your cardiovascular capacity. Both you and your horse will enjoy better fitness through a designed training program.

Physiology

Physiology is a branch of biology that deals with the functions and activities of living matter and of the physical and chemical phenomena involved. Your basic understanding of some simple physiology concepts will help you safely and effectively condition your horse.

Regardless of the type of activity your horse is engaged in, it should be gradually adjusting to longer and heavier workouts to prevent loss of fitness and to encourage an active increase in ability to perform and in the general physical and mental health of the horse. Fitness training and conditioning requires adaptations in the energy-generating processes of the horse's body as they affect the muscles, along with the supporting structures including bones, tendons and ligaments, metabolism, cardiovascular, temperature regulating, and the central nervous systems.

How the physiology of the horse adapts with training

An adequate period of physical conditioning based on your horse's current condition and level of activity will affect five important major systems including the cardiovascular, muscular, temperature regulating and central nervous systems along with the supporting structures including bones, tendons, ligaments which increase in the and/or strength during training. As the cardiovascular system improves in capacity to deliver oxygen to working muscles, the muscular system improves in its capacity to utilize oxygen. In addition, the temperature regulating system gains greater ability to lose body heat during exercise, while the central nervous system gains improved neuromuscular coordination enabling the horse to complete skills involved in a particular discipline more efficiently.

Although the amount of time it takes for a horse to gain a higher level of fitness will vary, the average time for structural and physiological adaptations to an effective exercise training program with an increase in oxygen delivery to muscles, increase in plasma volume and improved sweating response takes 1-2 weeks.

Conditioning principles

To achieve a conditioning and training effect, the horse must be subjected to gradual increases in workload with each new level of training being maintained until the body adapts to the additional stress. After the horse's body adapts to each new level of training, the workload is incrementally increased, again with a period of adaptation which is then followed by more intense training.

These alternate periods of increasing the workload and then allowing a period of adaptation is known as progressive loading. As the levels of exercise increase, the horse is gradually stressed to the point that it is able to tolerate the same exercise the next time with less stress. Both aerobic (occurring in the presence of oxygen) conditioning and anaerobic (occurring in the absence of oxygen) conditioning are involved in progressive loading.

For aerobic conditioning, progressive loading is accomplished through gradual increases in the duration and speed of the exercise on a weekly basis. For anaerobic conditioning, progressive loading is accomplished by a weekly increase in the exercise speed or in the number of repetitions of high intensity activity.

Sport-specific training

Training the horse to use the specific muscles and systems involved in the sport in which the horse competes, while considering the individual horse's fitness level, are two additional principles of conditioning to consider as you work with your horse. The specific muscles and systems involved in the discipline will be the focus of training.

Horses as individuals

Awareness of the individual differences in horses and the fact that their individual responses to conditioning will differ is another important principle of conditioning. The state of fitness at the beginning of a training program is extremely important. Age and prior activity level are important since some older horses have a reduced capacity to exercise, while younger horses are often capable of greater adaptations in response to training. To push an older horse or a horse that has been inactive for a long time into a full-scale training program without allowing for individual differences is to invite not only injury, but also mental and emotional resistance to the program.

Initial stage of conditioning

The appropriate frequency of exercise training will depend on the objectives of the training. When the objective is cardiovascular fitness, workouts performed 3 times a week on alternate days will allow time for tissue repair between workouts. One important fact that you should be aware of is that too frequent bouts of exercise are not likely to produce a faster conditioning response, and, may, in fact, predispose the horse to injury. Too little stress on tissues will not produce beneficial results, but too much stress or insufficient recovery time between exercise bouts will lead to a state of overtraining. Mild to severe muscle strains may occur and the supporting structures of limbs, bone, cartilage, ligaments and tendons that adapt more slowly to the stimulus of exercise may be compromised.

> ## Note
> ### Benefits to the horse
> Proper conditioning is a gift you can give your horse to ensure physical and mental health and well-being as his physiology changes and adapts to increasing levels of activity .

How do you know when your horse is "fit?"

The information that can be gained by monitoring your horse's heart rate is perhaps the best and most practical means of judging work effort. Monitoring the heart rate during exercise and recovery after exercise will give you a clear indication of your horse's fitness.

Together, these two heart rates are a means to quantify work effort and, over a period of time, show the progress the horse is making toward fitness. Strenuous workouts or faster running speeds will produce higher heart rates as fitness training takes place, especially in the early days of training. As the horse becomes more fit, the heart rate decreases during exercise. By keeping records of the heart rates, both during exercise and during recovery you will be able to compare the changing heart rates as your horse becomes more fit.

You can determine the heart rate by palpitating an arterial pulse, listening to the heart sounds with a stethoscope or by using a heart rate monitor. Since the heart rate drops rapidly after exercise ends, palpation or auscultation of the heart rate by using a stethoscope will not accurately reflect the heart rate during exercise.

The advantage of a heart rate monitor is that it gives a continuous reading of the horse's heart rate before, during and after exercise. If you do not care to invest in a heart monitor, you can still assess your horse's heart rate before and after exercise. In a well-conditioned horse, the heart rate will be around 60 beats per minute after 10 minutes of recovery even following strenuous workouts. Heart rate is sensitive to a variety of environmental factors including temperature, work surface, and excitement level. Exercise heart rates increase during hot weather, or on more yielding surfaces, and also show slower recovery rates. Illness and lameness also affect the horse's heart rate, so if it is elevated above normal after standardized exercise, the horse should be evaluated further.

Loss of fitness

Another principle of conditioning is that when a horse is no longer in training, it loses fitness. This loss of fitness is known as detraining, and the rate at which cardiovascular fitness, musculoskeletal strength and suppleness are lost determines the time required to recondition the horse. It is best to maintain a baseline level of fitness at all times including at the end of the competitive season with cardiovascular workouts twice a week at a reduced intensity and duration. Maintaining a baseline level of fitness allows faster reconditioning the following season.

Summary of conditioning principles
- An adequate level of fitness is necessary for horses to reach their potential
- Progressive loading with a period of exercise followed by a period of adaptation works well in conditioning for fitness

- Performance is most effectively improved by training the specific muscles and systems involved in the horse's discipline
- It is important to remember that different tissues in the body vary in their rate of adaptation to exercise with the cardiovascular and muscular systems respond rapidly
- The supporting structures including bones, ligaments, tendons adapt more slowly over a period of months
- Each horse is an individual and progress will vary
- The changes in nutrient requirements should be carefully monitored and increases in energy dense feed made when necessary to maintain horse in peak condition
- Training programs should allow adequate time to condition all the body systems
- A baseline of fitness should be maintained during off-seasons and other times of layoff unless the horse is injured or so ill that exercise would be counter-productive.

The effects of conditioning

Proper conditioning is a gift you can give your horse to ensure physical and mental health and well-being. The horse's body adapts to the rigors of conditioning with incremental increases in the intensity and duration of exercise through energy-generating processes involved in muscle contraction. The horse's body adapts to training by strengthening and improving the physical systems to increase efficiency and productivity. The cardiovascular system improves in the capacity to deliver oxygen to working muscles at the same time the muscular system improves in its capacity to utilize oxygen. Bones, tendons, ligaments and muscles increase in size and strength and the temperature regulating system achieves greater ability to lose body heat thereby avoiding excessive increases in body temperature. Neuromuscular coordination improves as the central nervous system adapts to the new skills required for a particular discipline.

The equine cardiovascular system

Within two to three weeks of the beginning of a regular exercise program, the blood volume increases due to an increase in the number of red blood cells and the volume of plasma. This increase in plasma volume along with an increase in red blood cells and hemoglobin provides an increase in the oxygen carrying capacity of the blood. Over a period of

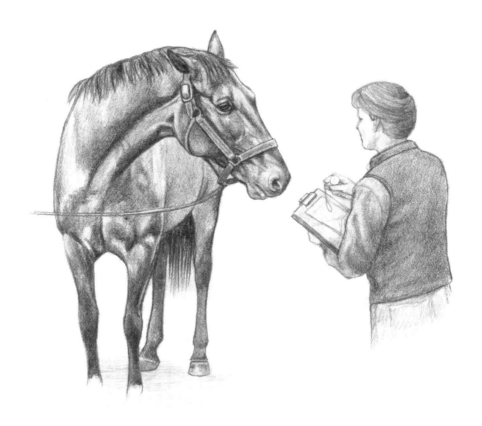

The equine athlete

Horses are amazing athletes. They are fleet and quick, and capable of sliding stops, spins and jumps despite weighing half a ton or more!

three to six months, an increase in the number of small blood vessels occurs within skeletal muscle increasing the transit time for blood through the muscle which improves the exchange of oxygen, glucose and fatty acids into the muscle and helps the muscle rid itself of carbon dioxide, lactic acid and heat.

Conditioning results in enlargement of the heart muscle enabling the heart to circulate blood more efficiently. This results in a reduction in heart rate at a given level of exercise since the heart is able to pump more blood with each beat and doesn't have to work as hard during exercise.

The recovery heart rate is also faster in well-trained horses, particularly endurance athletes.

The equine muscular system

A major component of the increase in cardiovascular capacity is the increase in the oxidative capacity of the muscles. The trained muscles are able to produce more energy because they are able to extract more oxygen from the blood. This allows a great proportion of energy to be produced by aerobic pathways early in the exercise period resulting in a delay of production of lactic acid and hydrogen ions that affect the muscle's ability to contract and prolonging the horse's capacity to work at a given intensity.

The supporting structures: bones, ligaments, tendons

Although relatively few studies have been done to examine how the horse's limbs adapt during training, it is known that the supporting structures adapt more slowly to training, taking up to six months before they sufficiently adapt. Recent studies have detected increases in bone density after four to five months of training. Because of the relatively slow adaptation of supporting structures to the exercise program, an incremental training program that gradually increases the length, speed and repetition of galloping is recommended to increase bone strength since the modeling response of bones is stimulated by fast work.

Recent research has found that the tendons and ligaments of mature horses have a limited ability to respond to training, but younger horses respond more readily. Although exercise training of horses less than two years old has been thought to be detrimental, the results of recent studies indicate the possibility that early training may enhance development of supporting structures of the limbs and perhaps reduce injury during training and competition. Always keep in mind, however, that a horse of any age should not be pushed beyond its physical limits. Supporting structures should be monitored closely during training. Each limb should be palpated for signs of swelling, heat and pain on a daily basis, and the training program should be adjusted accordingly.

Thermoregulatory adaptations of the horse

Research shows that the expansion of plasma volume that occurs within the first few weeks of training contributes to improved capacity for thermoregulation so that heat is dissipated and muscles can continue to receive the oxygen and fuels needed to sustain muscle contraction. Trained horses sweat earlier in the exercise bout than untrained horses showing that fit horses are able to remove excess heat before it overloads the thermoregulatory system. Horses that are not acclimated to warmer temperatures and high humidity need time to adjust to these conditions if they are to perform optimally.

It has been determined that a minimum of two weeks is necessary to acclimate a horse to performing in higher heat and humidity without detrimental effects. Merely exposing the horse to elevated heat and humidity will not cause adaptation to take place. Untrained horses take much longer to adapt to higher heat and humidity levels.

Neuromuscular coordination

Conditioning has a positive effect on the development of a horse's neuromuscular coordination and enables the horse to complete the skills required for a particular discipline. Schooling in a particular discipline develops the neuromuscular coordination and mental discipline necessary for participating in individual sporting activities such as dressage, eventing, reining, and cutting.

Neuromuscular coordination development is specific to each competitive sport, and a discussion of schooling techniques relative to the various sports is beyond the scope of this book.

Evaluating fitness - Establish a baseline

Before beginning a fitness training and conditioning program for your horse, it is important to establish the horse's baseline condition. This baseline condition is the starting point for your conditioning program to enhance and improve your horse's physical, mental, and emotional capabilities.

To make sure that the training and conditioning steps you take are effective and on track, you will need to do some record keeping by recording data and information about your horse's current condition, and then up-dating it daily or weekly as you progress through your program. Your record keeping should include a place to keep track of each of the horse's 7 vital signs including temperature, pulse rate, respiratory rate, capillary refill time, coloration of mucous membranes, level of hydration and gut sounds.

These vital signs, especially temperature, pulse rate, and respiratory rate tell a great deal about the condition of the cardiovascular, respiratory, muscular and thermoregulatory systems of your horse. You will also need to score your horse's body condition and record that information along with nutrition information including types of feed, amounts fed, and any adjustments you make to accommodate increasing physical demands. Keep anecdotal records related to any signs of illness, injury, or fatigue, appetite and water consumption, gait, attitude, and energy level as you monitor your horse's condition.

Make sure that your horse is up-to-date on vaccinations, deworming, hoof trimming, shoeing, and any other factors related to the horse's overall health and well being before beginning fitness training.

The following information will help you in not only determining the current condition of your horse for your baseline, but are also the steps you will take in doing a daily once-over to make sure your horse is in condition to continue with on-going exercise, training and conditioning.

Vital signs

Vital signs include body temperature, heart rate, respiratory rate - all noted as part of a regular physical exam. You should learn how to measure these vital signs, as wall as other important indicators of the horse's physical condition, including - capillary refill time, gut sounds, and mucous membrane color. See Your horse's vital signs in the General Care chapter for descriptions and instructions for measure these vital signs.

Body condition scoring

Body condition scoring is a systematic analysis of the amount of fat that occurs on a specific animal. It is used to determine that the nutrition level is satisfactory for the animal. An overweight or underweight animal will not condition well, and should first be brought to a body condition score of 5 or 6 before serious training. Learn how to body condition score in Chapter 5, General Care.

Heat, inflammation and gait

Now that you have determined your horse's vital signs and body conditioning score, you will want to observe and check out how well the muscular system of the horse is working and note any signs of injury, strain, or lack of limb coordination.

This can be done in 4 steps as your horse stands on hard level ground.

1) Begin by walking around your horse starting on one side with the head, neck, body, hip, legs and then check out the other side in the same way. Look and feel for any signs of injuries, bumps, bruises or tense spots. Run your hands over the limbs and hoofs to check for variations in temperature or heat that might indicate inflammation.

2) Next, jog your horse around in a small circle on the end of a lead rope to observe the movements of the horse's shoulders, head, its tail position, and how the horse moves. Watch for favoring of any shoulder or limb, and for a nodding of the head that indicates a hoof or leg-related lameness. Notice how the horse carries its tail to see how it travels in relationship to how it moved on preceding days. Note inconsistencies in hoof patterns. If a horse is feeling pain in its body, it often shows up as a change in the hoof pattern, in which case you will explore the horse's limbs with flexion tests and palpitation of any areas that appear to be painful or inflamed.

Using your hands, carefully palpitate along the sides of the horse's spine to check for sore spots, especially in the loin and muscles along the croup. Begin at the poll on the left side and press your fingertips firmly, but gently in a slow continuous sweep from the top of the horse's head along the spine's length checking the neck, withers, back and croup to the base of the tail. Message any tender spots to relax bunched muscles.

3) Now, check the flexion of the knees, ankles, shoulders, stifles and hocks. You will most likely need to have someone hold the horse or you can hold the end of the lead, being careful to keep it away from the horse's feet. Flexions can be hard for some horses, so be careful and if the horse is agitated or too reluctant, don't force the issue.

Begin by picking up the left front hoof as if you are going to clean it, then fold the horse's leg up, bracing the horse's knee just above your locked knees.

With both hands on the ankle, exert pressure on the knee joint by pulling the cannon bone and fetlock towards the horse's elbow, checking for flexibility and observing any flinching response by the horse.

To check the ankle or fetlock, move your hands down to the horse's toe and pull the toe firmly towards your waist, putting flex on the ankle joint and again checking for sensitivity and flexibility.

4) Next, unfold the horse's knee joint and carefully pull the horse's foreleg first back toward the tail and finally straight out in front of the horse to check the shoulder for soreness, range of motion and flexibility.

Repeat the flexions on the horse's right side, looking for change from the previous day and comparing the horse's reactions with its normal responses.

To check hocks and stifles on hind legs, face forward and hold the horse's hoof up high for at least 60 seconds to compress the hock, then have an assistant immediately trot the horse forward.

Since this flexion requires a helper, you may not do it every day, but it should be considered necessary if the horse appears to be developing a hock problem.

By going through these steps, you will be able to methodically examine the horse's body for injury or muscle soreness. After you've done these checks a few times, you will get to know your horse well enough to quickly detect any problems or changes.

Daily workout

Daily exercise is essential for the over-all health of your horse. A daily workout benefits your horse in the following ways:

- It increases the horse's stamina and endurance
- It improves the functioning of the heart and lungs
- It enhances the functioning of muscles, tendons and ligaments.

Daily exercise aids motility of the digestive tract and allows the horse to clear out secretions from the lungs as it breathes more deeply during exercise than when simply standing around.

In addition, exercise helps prevent behavior problems associated with confinement and boredom. The horse becomes more mentally alert while interacting with a handler and this leads to quicker reflexes and better coordination. As part of your horse's fitness and conditioning, the daily workout give you the opportunity to work with your equine buddy in ways that will not only improve the physical and mental health of your horse, but will also improve your health and certainly your working relationship with your horse.

It is important to take a look at the horse's physical condition before beginning an exercise program and then to ease into the program. By monitoring the horse's condition before and after each workout, you will have a good idea of how well your workout program is progressing. If the horse is young or older, isn't used to much physical activity, or has health problems, you will need to start with light exercise and gradually work up to a level that will either maintain or improve the horse's level of fitness. If you have questions about how much exercise your horse needs, talk

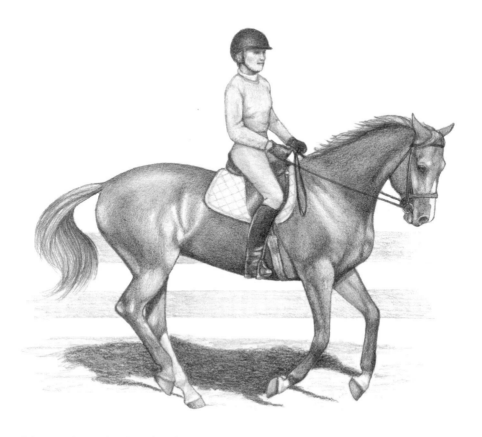

Mental and physical

Every time you work with your horse, you are developing his physical and mental capabilities. Proper feeding and exercise result in both better health and increased safety.

with your veterinarian about developing a good daily workout regimen.

Basic elements of a daily workout

It is helpful to think of a workout as consisting of three phases: Warm up. Work out. Cool down. These three phases should precede each ride. Doing so will reduce the chance of injury, provide a period of focused activity and learning, and end with a calming period that helps the horse and rider to bond as a team.

Warming up your horse

Warming up is essential for getting the best performance and for reducing the chance of injuries. It involves a gradual increase in exercise intensity so that the limbs move freely, the horse relaxes mentally, and there is increased oxygen delivery to the muscles which enhances their ability to work aerobically and reduces lactate build up.

A number of different activities can be used for warming up your horse. In fact, any light physical exercise that gets the horse's musculoskeletal system working can serve as a warm-up depending on the age and condition of the horse. Allowing the horse to walk or trot at a nice, easy pace for 10 - 15 minutes works well for most horses Longeing the horse at an easy pace to get it moving and the muscles active works well also. If the horse has turn-out time in the pasture before beginning the daily workout, that will serve part of the warm-up.

The air temperature needs to be taken into consideration during the warm up. During cold weather, it will take longer for muscles to reach their ideal working temperature. A warming blanket or a heat lamp may be used during cold weather to warm the muscles prior to exercise. After 5-10 minutes of warm-up activity, the musculoskeletal system should be warm enough to do some stretching and some suppling exercises.

Suppling exercises

A regular stretching routine is good insurance against injury and enhances sensory nerve endings in muscles, tendons, ligaments and joints that give the horse's brain information about movement and body position. Suppling exercises increase your horse's suppleness and elasticity, and greatly reduce the chances of pulled muscles or tendons. In addition, stretching and suppling exercises improve circulation and help relieve pain, inflammation and muscle spasms.

Suppling exercises fall into three categories: dynamic, passive or natural. Natural suppling exercises include activities the horse does naturally such as rolling, grazing, scratching and biting at flies. As the horse engages in each of these activities, flexibility and suppleness are maintained and improved. Passive suppling exercises are usually done prior to riding and after riding while the horse is warmed up. In effect, passive suppling exercises consist of stretching the horse's shoulders, hips, back, neck and poll and can play an important role in symmetrical development. Effective passive suppling exercises include moving the hind leg forward and across the body under the widest part of the stomach; folding the foreleg and rotating the point of the shoulder up and forward, stretching the neck forward and down between the horse's knees and to the side towards the girth area.

Dynamic suppling exercises are accomplished by either riding or walking the horse through a series of traditional suppling exercises including turns, circles, serpentines, doing lateral work, making transitions forward and backward, and leg yielding. As the horse becomes accustomed to the dynamic suppling exercises, include smaller circles and add more difficult lateral movements. The purpose of suppling exercises is to systematically get the horse's musculoskeletal system working together to develop suppleness and flexibility throughout the body.

Working out

Horses that are pastured and free to move around most or all of the day will benefit from a 15 to 20 minute workout each day. Horses that are stabled most of the time will require at least a 30 minute workout each day and will benefit most from an hour or more of exercise activity. Competitive horses are normally worked for an hour each day, five days a week. Depending on your horse's workload and whether or not your horse is a performance or competition horse, your daily workout will be specific to the kind of work your horse does. The daily workout helps condition your horse for the type of work it does.

Although riding is viewed by many as the best way to exercise your horse, you can vary the routine by longeing the horse. Longeing works well with horses that cannot be ridden for whatever reason and in young horses, longeing may be sufficient to initiate cardiovascular adaptations. The workload during longeing may be increased by working the horse with more impulsion or on a deeper surface such as a bed of sand. When a horse canters on a loose deep surface the heart rate is around 180 beats per minute and a significant elevation of blood lactate occurs. If you are doing longeing on a loose, deep surface for conditioning, introduce the work slowly with gradual increments to avoid muscular or tendon injuries.

Cooling your horse down

The way you approach cooling down your horse will depend on the weather and other environmental conditions. Following the workout, a period of relaxed walking will help the horse adjust to lowered activity. The main goal of the cool-down period is to get the horse to a point where it is, cool, dry, and relaxed, but not cold. If temperatures are cold, a blanket to help maintain body heat will be necessary once the horse's temperature and heart rate are back to normal. If the weather is hot and the horse is overheated, it should be moved to a shady area, and, if necessary the horse may be sponged or sprayed with cool water to enhance heat loss. The horse can be offered small drinks of water to replace fluids lost during exercise. No hay or feed should be offered until the horse's temperature is below 102 degrees F. to minimize the risk of colic. A little hay is safe feed at that point, but grain should be saved until later.

Consistency of exercise

Whatever form of exercise you choose for your horse's daily workout, it is important to be consistent in maintaining the daily schedule. Irregular exercise predisposes some horses to "tying up" and injuries can occur when a horse is given time off and then brought back into a full daily workout program without time for retraining

Suppleness and flexibility

The terms "suppleness" and "flexibility" mean essentially the same thing, but each has a slightly different connotation as used in relationship to exercise of the horse's body. Flexibility indicates the ability to bend without breaking, and suppleness indicates easy movement that flows from one muscle to the next and from tendon to ligament to muscle without creating stress or strain on any one part. As research has shown, muscles are suppled and strengthened by alternation between contracting them actively and then stretching them passively by contracting the antagonistic muscles.

As the muscles are suppled and strengthened, the musculoskeletal system of the horse becomes more finely interconnected and by doing so, bones, tendons, ligaments, and muscles work together more coherently without undue stress on any one part of the system.

The rider is an additional component in the suppleness and flexibility of the horse. Even the most well-trained and supple horse will become stiff under a rider who does not align and center her body correctly in the saddle or doesn't use the reins and her hands correctly. A riders stiffness, lopsidedness or tension often results in the same symptoms in the horse, and until the rider identifies and corrects those trouble spots, the horse will remain confused, tense and stiff to some degree.

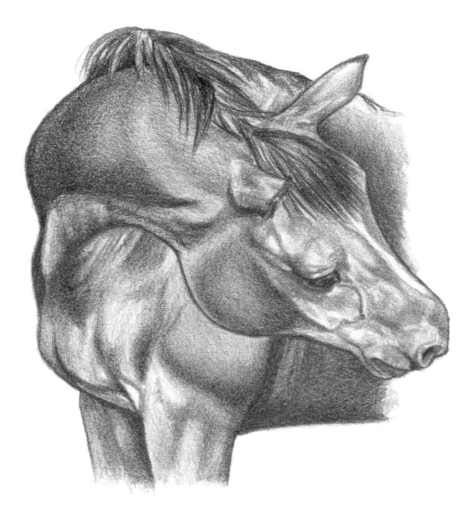

Passive suppling

Horses can be encouraged to passively stretch to obtain a hand-fed treat.
Dynamic suppling, where the trainer actively manipulates joints should not be
performed without training.

Endurance training

Training for improved endurance is focused on improving the aerobic
conditioning of the horse. Endurance is the ability to maintain a high level
of work before muscular fatigue occurs. When formulating an endurance
training program, it is important to emphasize activities that improve the

cardiovascular efficiency as well as the development of muscle strength required for climbing and descending hills.

Long and slow can be used to characterize endurance training. Over a period of time, the horse is exercised for progressively longer periods of low to moderate heart-rate activities. In general, speed control is used to maintain the animal in an aerobic state, allowing the development of cardiovascular efficiency.

Endurance training - The process

Endurance training relies on the low intensity aerobics exercise that is called Long Slow Distance (LSD). The goal is to improve the efficiency of both the cardiovascular system, as well as the metabolic efficiency associated with muscles, and supporting structures.

The process depends on exercising all of the horse's gaits at a relatively slow speed for longer and longer distances. The walk, trot and canter are all worked, ideally combining arena and trail work. Depending on the age, breed and previous experience, it may take from 3 to 12 months to reach a level of cardiovascular and metabolic fitness for endurance type activities.

General rules

Young horses should not be worked more than 3 or 4 days a week during the development of basic endurance. The objective is to obtain a basic level of fitness that prepares the horse to cope with easy exercise of walking, trotting and cantering for a period of one hour at an average speed for 4 to 5 miles per hour (6 to 8 kilometers per hour). This includes 2 to 3 minutes of cantering while maintaining a heart rate of less than 160 beats per minute.

Intensity

Keeping intensity low to moderate is very important during the early stages of training. Continuous movement is also important at the early stages. For more advanced training interval training techniques can be used to improve overall strength.

Duration

Start with 15 to 20 minute training sessions for the young or unconditioned horse. Divide the early training sessions with most time spent on brisk walking, followed by time spent trotting and no cantering. After a period, decrease the time walking in favor of more trotting and cantering. Keep the speed low, and monitor heart rate to assure that the horse is staying in an aerobic condition (less than 160 beats per minute).

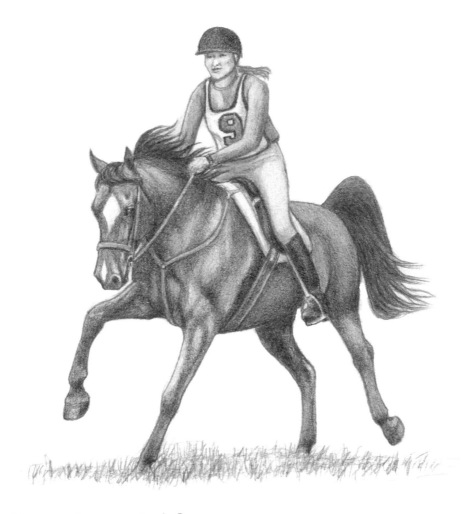

Why endurance train?

All horses benefit from endurance exercises and trail riding as part of over-all horse training. Endurance training is especially useful for horses that are anxious or spooky.

Add 5 minutes every week, until you are able to meet the objectives set above. At this point, your horse has a level of conditioning that is appropriate for any horse considered fit.

Strength training

Strength, power, and endurance are the three major components of any athletic goal: Strength as it relates to the training of horses is the ability of the horse to produce and apply force, while power is the rate of force generation. When formulating a strength training program for your horse, it is important to determine whether the primary requirement in the muscles is for power or for endurance. This will depend on the particular sport or competition in which your horse will be engaged.

A successful strength training program is based on knowledge of the movements and muscular actions involved in the sport so that exercises will simulate the range and speed of motion used in the competition.

> ## Note
> ### Heart rate recovery
>
> Heart rate recovery is an excellent indicator of fitness. Following a period of measured exercise, note the amount of time it takes for the heart rate to return to a normalized level, normally 80 beats per minute. Equine heart rate monitors are available to easily measure the recovery time.

As a component of muscular fitness, improvement in muscular strength in the muscles not only enhances performance, but also reduces injuries by stabilizing the joints and preventing muscle strains.

The process

Four variables affect the strength training process. First, the force of muscle contractions needs to be considered. Second, the speed of movement will affect the outcomes of strength training. Third, the number of repetitions you put your horse through will have a strong influence on how rapidly the strength training progresses, and lastly, the frequency of workouts will help determine how rapidly and well the process works.

General rules

For the exercises to be effective, they should be specific for the muscle groups and for the type of contractions used in the competitions or the work that the horse does. In addition, for effective training, the trainer needs to be aware that low intensity exercise cannot prepare the muscles for high intensity athletic performance and should adjust the exercises accordingly.

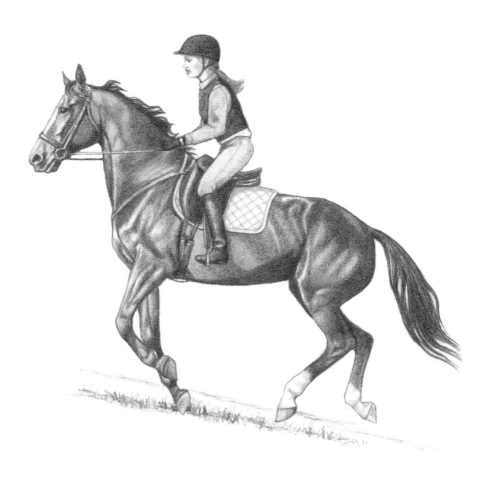

Use of terrain

Terrain can be used to develop different aspects of your horse's physiology. For example, cantering up hills is very effective for developing a powerful hindquarter.

Intensity

Since the force of the contraction is the most important variable in strength training, carrying or pulling more weight, working on steeper hills or jumping higher fences are the kinds of activities that provide the most benefit in strength training. Also, the speed of the movement should be the same as the speed of the actual sport to give the horse the maximum benefit from the exercise.

115

Duration

Research shows that relatively short sessions of approximately 20 minutes work well when training for strength. The number of repetitions of the exercise movements are more important than the length of time spent. Research shows that it is best not to work a horse to the point of exhaustion because of the vulnerability of the tendons, ligaments and supporting muscles. When signs of fatigue appear, it is best to stop strenuous work and begin the cool down to avoid the danger of injury.

Methods of strength training

Generally, conditioning on a loose, deep surface and riding through snow or water, helps strengthen specific muscle groups, while also increasing cardiovascular loading and encouraging active joint flexion through a wide range of motion. The use of gradients on hills or other terrain is an outstanding way of strength training your equine. Using gradients can be approached from several different angles and all gaits can be used, thereby providing a variety of strength-building activities. Trotting exercises on a moderate incline are especially beneficial to endurance horses that will encounter on gradients during competitions. Gradual downhill work is beneficial for sports that require a high degree of collection.

Working through a series of forward movements, halting, and reining back on a downhill gradient improves both strength and balance. Downhill conditioning at a trot or canter is good exercise for horses that are being prepared for eventing, combined driving and endurance racing. Because this type of exercise creates stress on joints, it should be limited.

Factors that affect progress

Horses need cardiovascular and muscular endurance to be able to perform in equestrian sports such as eventing, jumping, and endurance. In the long run, every horse benefits from a good exercise program that develops the necessary endurance for the horse's workload. Training involves many hours and many miles on the trail, usually maintaining either a trot or a canter with occasional walking when the terrain dictates slowing down. Rarely is there an all-out gallop, as in Thoroughbred racing.

Conclusion

The natural horse moves almost constantly, 20 hours a day. Survival is conditioned on being able to evade or outrun the predator. Horses in the natural setting are very well conditioned.

As we move our horses into a captive setting, the ability to wander and move becomes limited. The nature of feeding horses in most settings does not promote movement, and often results in a horse that is overweight and poorly conditioned.

In this chapter, you learned the basics of physiology that relate to horse conditioning. You now understand how important it is to the horse's physical and mental condition to provide consistent exercise. You also understand the need for measuring the progress of an exercise program, and are now equipped to use body condition scoring and vital sign recording to chart the fitness progress of your horse.

Horse's enjoy work, and are amazingly willing to work with you in the development of some highly sophisticated skills that make horsemanship an ever-challenging pursuit. If you are a goal oriented person, this part of horse ownership may prove to be one of the most rewarding.

Top-5 takeaways

1. Horses are naturally active, and need physical exercise as part of their daily lives. For most horse owners, turnout is the most feasible method to provide the opportunity for exercise.

2. Horses are natural athletes, they are capable of both explosive powerful sprints as well as slow and long endurance rides. In both cases, the horse must be conditioned over a period of time, or the chances of injury are increased.

3. Every workout should be divided into a warm-up period, a period of physical and mental exercise, and a cool-down period. 15 minutes of warm-up, 30 minutes of actual training, and 15 minutes of warm-down are a typical session.

4. Body condition scoring is an objective method of appraising your feeding program. Shoot for a score of 5 or 6 for working horses, and you may need a grain supplement to maintain this score.

5. Getting your horse fit and conditioned has the additional benefit of providing better fitness and conditioning for you!

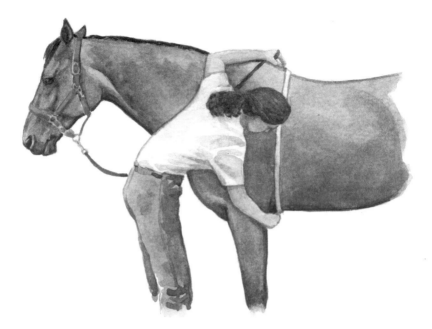

Chapter 4 General care

Introduction

If you read only one chapter in this book from start to finish, this chapter on general care should be it. Your understanding and implementation of the basic care activities outlined in this chapter will result in a healthier and happier horse, and you will also save money by avoiding veterinary bills that result from not getting the basics right.

General care is focused on prevention of disease. Basic vaccinations and parasite control should be a routine event on your annual health calendar. These relatively simple tasks will save you money and potentially heartache by avoiding some really nasty and potentially fatal diseases.

General care is also all about proper nutrition. Unbalanced or improper feeding can lead to a host of conditions, especially in older horses. In many cases, a horse does not have access to large pasture areas and relies on the owner for the majority of its food. How much to feed? What to feed? When to feed? You will probably be surprised at the answers at first, but then in thinking about the natural horse it will all make sense.

This chapter touches on essential information that is developed in more detail in other chapters. For example, a healthy horse depends on the animals physical condition, and opportunities to reduce stress through physical activity. We devote a chapter to fitness and conditioning, because it is important to the overall wellbeing of the horse.

We also stress the daily care that your horse deserves. Attention to body condition, noting the invariable scrapes and cuts, observing minor lameness or changes in feeding patterns that may predict a colic. Through daily observation and care, you will become an expert in sensing when something is wrong - prior to it becoming a bigger problem.

This chapter will also prepare you for the inevitable health issues that arise as your horse enters his senior years. Changes in diet, condition and health for the senior horse requires additional care and knowledge of the horse owner.

Five main areas of preventive care

- Vaccinations
- Worming
- Hoof care
- Dental care
- Daily care

Each of these areas has a special significance in the health of your horse. Dental care and hoof care are so important that we have chapters dedicated to these two elements of horse healthcare.

Vaccinations

An effective equine vaccination program always begins with a discussion with your veterinarian. However, with rapid developments in vaccine technology and a seemingly endless array of products on the market, it is often difficult to know exactly what will work best for a

Watch this
How to vaccinate your horse

Most people become very comfortable providing the vaccinations that are required to protect your horse against some very nasty diseases. A short video is provided that will help you learn how to, and gain confidence with, vaccinating your own horse. Access this video by entering the following URL into your browser:

https://horse-health-matters.com/videos/vaccinate-your-horse

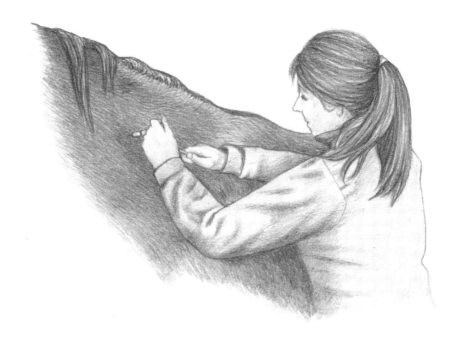

Do it yourself

Vaccinations and worming are two activities that you can easily perform. Ask your veterinarian to show you how and order vaccines and anthelmintics (dewormers) online for greater savings.

horse in any given circumstances. This is where the advice of a knowledgeable veterinarian is of crucial importance because vaccines can be costly and if not given appropriately can have negative consequences for the horse. In some cases, you may depend on your veterinarian to vaccinate your horse, but you may also want to do at least some of the vaccinations yourself following the directions of your vet. Because your horse needs periodic booster shots in many cases, as well as other shots, having syringes and other supplies available to administer vaccines can help ensure that your horse receives needed immunizations and booster shots in a timely fashion.

By seeking the advice of your veterinarian about which vaccines are important, not only will you save money on vaccines and vet bills, but the health of your horse will be better maintained.

Diseases against which horses are vaccinated fall into two main categories as defined by the American Association of Equine Practitioners (AAEP): core vaccinations and risk-based vaccinations. For horses with a solid vaccination history, the AAEP guidelines are fairly straight forward. Core vaccinations "Protect against diseases that are endemic to a region, those with potential public health significance, required by law, virulent/highly infectious, and/or those posing a risk of severe disease."

"Core vaccines have clearly demonstrated efficacy and safety, and exhibit a high enough level of patient benefit and low enough level of risk to justify their use in all equids." In other words, core vaccines are a safe way to protect horses against dangerous diseases that carry a high risk of exposure.

Core diseases in horses include Eastern and Western equine encephalitis, West Nile virus and rabies.

In addition, to core diseases, a number of serious diseases are considered risk based diseases. Some horses may be at higher risk of particular diseases by virtue of age, geography, housing, or function. Vaccines against diseases in this category may vary in efficacy or risk of complication. Also, not every horse will be exposed to every disease. Risk-based disease vaccination planning requires the input of a veterinarian familiar with your horse, its use and where you live

Risk based diseases include equine-herpes virus, influenza, strangles, Potomac horse fever, Venezuelan equine encephalomyelitis, equine viral arteritis, Hendra virus, and botulism.

In some cases, your veterinarian may recommend other vaccinations based on the condition of your horse and the exposure to disease threats. These special risk situations include newborn foals in which the immune system initially has very limited function.

In the weeks after birth, almost all of the foal's ability to fight disease comes from the antibodies it gained from the mare (see above). As the mare's antibodies wane, the foal's immune system "comes on-line." However, one set of shots at weaning is not generally sufficient to properly protect a foal against disease. With a few exceptions, vaccination requires repeated exposure to generate immunity. With foals we talk about a primary "vaccination series." It is important not to skimp on these vaccinations. Though no one likes the idea of giving multiple shots to a young horse, there is evidence to suggest that the quality of early immunization can impact a horse's immunity to disease throughout life. It is much safer to bite the bullet and comply with the entire foal vaccination series rather than to risk immune failure later.

Vaccination success relies upon repeat exposure. With a few exceptions specific to some of the newer vaccines, vaccination works by exposing the immune system to a small amount of a protein specific to the disease causing organism (the antigen.) The first exposure to the antigen primes the immune system. However, the disease-fighting antibodies do not develop significantly until the body encounters the antigen a second or third time.

Adult horses that have never been vaccinated or where vaccination history is unknown (i.e. auction purchase, rescue, etc.) will require an initial vaccination series similar to that for a foal.

Making sure the vaccines you use are not out-dated and are administered in the correct dosage via the correct route, either intravenous or intramuscular, or in some cases, orally is very important

Parasites

One of the keys to good horse health is a regularly scheduled deworming program that is followed year in and year out, but is kept up to date based on the latest and best information available about what works and doesn't work when it comes to ridding your horse of parasites. Equine parasites are with us every day of the year, as they lay eggs that hatch into larvae that turn into adult worms that start the process all over again. During their passage through the horse's system, worms injure organ systems and create problems that lead to anemia, diarrhea, weight loss, nutritional deficiencies, and other conditions that jeopardize the life of your horse. In addition, researchers estimate that worms are a predisposing factor in 90 percent of cases of intestinal colic.

> ## Watch this
> ### How to deworm your horse
> Visit this books website to learn more about deworming your horse. A short video is provided that will help you learn how to, and gain confidence with, deworming your own horse. Access this video by entering the following URL into your browser:
>
> https://horse-health-matters.com/videos/deworm-your-horse

Fortunately, dewormers rank very high in medical advancements made over the last few years, and horses, in general, are healthier as a result. When things go well, it's easy to become complacent about the routines that have taken us this far. Don't let that happen to you when it comes to the important strategies of an effective deworming program. Working with your veterinarian it is important to establish the worming program and environmental control practices that will work best for your horse. Once your program is established, it is important to keep a supply of the necessary dewormers in your barn or tack room to be used on schedule following the directions given by your veterinarian.

Facts about parasites/worms

Many parasites can take a toll on your horses systems causing illness, loss of productivity, and general deterioration of the horse's health and include:

- Large Strongyles (Bloodworms): Infection rate is between 70 and 100 percent of all horses. These parasites can destroy arterial walls, blood vessels, impair circulation, and lead to colic, anemia, diarrhea, fever, poor condition, brain damage, and other disorders.
- Larvae of small strongyles penetrate the walls of the horse's intestine, where they encyst, leading to inflammation that results in anorexia, weight loss, and chronic colic. When the larvae emerge from the gut wall in spring or in times of stress, they cause severe diarrhea.
- Ascarids, also known as roundworms, grow up to 12 inches in length, can cause colic, heart damage, liver and lung damage, and, in older horses and foals, can injure the intestines.
- Stomach bots infect nearly all horses. Eggs are deposited on hairs near the mouth and hatch into larvae, which find their way into the mouth. They burrow into pockets between the molar teeth, causing dental disease, are swallowed, and then attach themselves to the lining of the stomach where they cause irritations, ulcerations, and perforations of the stomach wall.
- Pinworms cause intense anal itching, leading to attempts by the horse to decrease the itching by rubbing its tail and hindquarters against a post or wall, eventually damaging the hair, skin, and tail. A large number of pinworms can cause inflammation of the colon and episodes of colic.
- Large tape worms are extremely common in some areas of the world. The can affect both horses and humans and may cause

severe ulcerations of the large intestine if left untreated.

- Stomach worms, also known as Habronema cause the larval attacks that cause summer sores on the skin and conjunctivitis in the eyes of horses. These small worms live in colonies in the wall of the stomach and can produce severe gastritis and, in some cases, tumor-like enlargements in the stomach wall. If the stomach wall ruptures, peritonitis may occur. Hairworms or small stomach worms can produce severe infestations that cause gastritis, with ulcers, weight loss, and anemia.

Parasite control

It is important to work with your veterinarian who can help you determine which kinds of parasites are most likely to infest your horse. Your vet can help you determine what kind of schedule and which deworming products will work best for you and your horse in your particular circumstances. A "purge" or interval program works by breaking the cycle in the parasite's life, essentially killing the adult worms before

> **Note**
> ## Strategic vs. rotational worming
> Many veterinarians, fearful of resistant parasites due to over-medicating, are encouraging strategic worming. Instead of rotating wormers. Strategic worming includes testing and treatment of animals that are parasite carriers.

they can lay eggs. By reducing the number of eggs, the exposure to parasites is minimized, unless the horse is pastured or around other horses that are on less-than-effective deworming programs.

A daily program works by killing the early-stage larvae your horse gets in his mouth before they penetrate body tissues. By killing the larvae before they begin migrating, internal parasite levels are minimized, even if the environment is heavily infested or out of your control. Whether you choose a purge program or a daily deworming program, you will need to take steps to target the other parasites that are not adequately controlled with your chosen program. These include bots, tapeworms, and encysted small strongyles.

The three classes of anthelmintic or parasiticide drugs are Benzimidazoles, Macrocyclic lactone, and Tetra hydro-pyrimidine. Each has strengths and weaknesses, and it is necessary to switch deworming agents periodically to prevent the worms from becoming immune to one dewormer. Also, different formulas kill different kinds of worms, so it's important to rotate the dewormers to be sure to kill all kinds of worms.

In general, deworming agents will never be completely effective in ridding a horse of parasites because of the continuing problem of reinfection, the impossibility of killing all parasites as they go through different stages or become encysted, and the development of drug-resistant worms, especially in the case of small strongyles that have become resistant to the drug class, Benzimidazoles. For effectiveness, environmental control of parasites must be an integral part of your deworming management program by picking up and disposing of manure in pastures at least twice a week. Mow pastures regularly to break up manure piles and expose parasite eggs and larvae to the elements. When possible rotate pastures and allow sheep and cattle to graze intermittently to interrupt the life cycles of parasites.

Horse owners should also realize that at times, a horse will act as if it doesn't feel well after being dewormed and it will become lethargic. Several theories are suggested as to the cause of this including a reaction to a heavy parasite load being killed, or the emergence of large numbers of encysted small strongyle larvae stressing the horse's system. If your horse is lethargic or shows symptoms of illness after deworming, check with your veterinarian as to possible causes. A thorough deworming program, combined with environmental control, will go a long way toward making sure your horse's health, appearance, performance and comfort are maximized in every way.

Dental Care

The field of dental care in horses is rapidly expanding. Increasingly people are becoming aware of the importance of regular maintenance of a horse's mouth, not only for ensuring efficient feed utilization but for continued performance. In young horses dental check-ups should be performed every six monthly to ensure corrections are performed before they cause a major problem with discomfort especially related to the bit. It is important to have a thorough dental examination performed before a young horse is broken in. This is the time when they are introduced to the bit and bridle and also a time that many changes are occurring with the teeth.

Pain from sharp enamel points or loose caps can cause problems in training if the horse is distracted by mouth pain and doesn't respond appropriately. 'Bit seating' which is rounding of the front edge of the front cheek teeth can greatly improve ridden behavior in some horses.

According to Angela Hawker, DVM, of Cambridge Equine Hospital, a common misconception is that there will be some outward sign of a dental problem. By the time a horse starts to lose weight, drop feed or show other signs, the problem can be quite advanced.

If your horse's teeth are regularly floated and cared

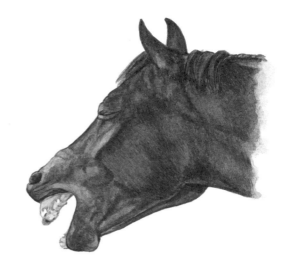

Equine dental care explained

Learn more about equine dental care in Chapter 2. Ignoring your horse's teeth is a common occurance for new horse owners.

for, most dental problems will be avoided. Depending on your horse's diet, hardness of teeth, and jaw alignment, floating may be necessary on an annual basis, depending on what your veterinarian/dentist prescribes. Talking to your equine dentist or veterinarian for instructions on how you can examine your horses teeth can be very beneficial, both to your horse and your pocket book.

Once you know how to do it, you can make sure you check your horse's teeth on a regular basis. By noticing any changes in dental surfaces or eating habits, you can be proactive in making sure your horse gets needed dental care. By taking the time and making the effort, you will avoid complications that could affect your horse's health and vitality, as well as the enjoyment you get from your horse.

One Word of Caution: Do not attempt to reach into your horse's mouth and feel the teeth unless you have been taught safe methods for doing so. The horse may bite, or you may shred your fingers on a sharp edge or point of a tooth. To learn more about caring for your horse's teeth and mouth, read the chapter on Dental Care.

Hoof Care

Getting to know your horse's hoofs by making sure that the hoofs are picked and cleaned on a regular basis, usually before and after each ride, or at least a couple of times a week is a very important part of preventive care in maintaining good horse health. While picking out any small rocks or objects, pay attention to what is going on with each hoof. Is the temperature and pulse normal? Does the frog have a firm texture, without any indication of problems? Note any signs of injury, including punctures. Sniff the horse's feet to make sure that no bad odors indicating thrush or other infections are present. In addition to making sure the horse's hoofs are picked, cleaned and checked on a regular basis, your horse's diet should provide for the best possible hoof health. Check with your veterinarian or farrier to see if the diet is adequate or if a change in feed or the addition of supplements would be helpful.

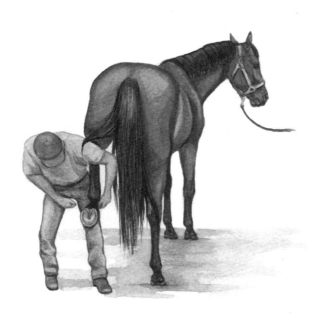

Hoof care explained

Hoof care is so important that we devote an entire chapter on it. See Chapter 7.

If your horse is shod, check the shoes on a regular basis, even if the horse is more of a pasture ornament and isn't ridden often, make sure all nails are in the correct position and that the shoe isn't loose, pulling away, or shifting position. Call the farrier whenever you see problems with the shoes. If you are hauling the horse to shows, events, or for trail rides, protect the horse's hoofs by using proper bandages or boots. Several good options are available, including bandages and boots with Velcro fasteners for easy application and removal.

Don't allow your horse to spend time standing in mud, wet grass, boggy pasture, or unsanitary, urine-soaked bedding. These conditions lead to swelling, softening of the hoofs, and infections such as thrush. When wet conditions are followed by dry conditions, the hoofs will split or crack, leading to discomfort and infections that may lead to abscesses causing lameness. Work with your farrier by scheduling regular visits. Once a farrier gets to know the horse's needs, a timetable of visits can be worked out to make sure hoof health is an ongoing priority. In many cases, a capable farrier will be willing to instruct you in day-to-day care of the hoofs and shoes to maximize care without straining your budget or time schedule. Learn more about the well being of your horse's hoofs by reading the Chapter on Hoof Care

Daily care

Most horse owners realize that a horse's well-being requires physical, emotional and social necessities that are a part of the natural needs of their species. Creating a natural environment as close to a horse's natural lifestyle as possible helps domesticated horses live a more natural life. In the horse's natural environment, intellectual stimulation arises from everyday tasks and interactions with other horses in the herd. Horses are intelligent and social creatures. As such, they require more than just physical necessities such as food and shelter, but also mental stimulation. Failure to provide these will affect the horse's mental and emotional health. In turn, this will eventually result in the development of behavioral issues or bad habits which can be destructive to their surroundings, their health, and their riding performance.

Your domesticated horse needs care and attention in the following areas on a daily basis for maximum well being:
- Feed and water
- Exercise and physical conditioning
- Grooming along with a daily once-over
- Shelter and a quiet environment
- Socialization and companionship

Feeding and watering

Feed is very important to horses since nature designed their systems to spend much of their day grazing, chewing, swallowing and digesting their feed. Hay and other roughages provide nutrients and satiety for your horse. On average, a horse must consume about two percent of its body weight per day to maintain body weight and digestive health. Different ages, classes and workloads of horses require different levels of nutrients from the hay they eat. A combination of these and other factors make choosing the right type of hay for your horse a challenge, but with a little consideration, you as a horse owner are in a position to analyze and compare and make the best choice for your particular horse.

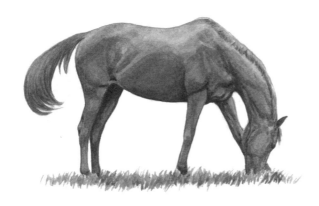

Equine nutrition explained

You will spend more money on feeding your horse than for anything else. Learn the fundamentals will assure a healthy and happy horse - and save you money. Learn more in Chapter 9

If you are fortunate enough to have a good pasture where your horse can forage, you are in luck. If not, as a responsible horse owner, you may want to have a hay analysis on the hay you are feeding your horse. A hay analysis gives the level of crude protein, total digestible nutrients, calcium, phosphorus, magnesium and potassium in the hay so you can make wise hay buying decisions.

A diet of high quality hay or grass will provide the energy and protein that a non-working horse requires. Remember that there are big differences between legume hay such as alfalfa and clover and grass-type hays such as Bermuda and Timothy. Consider giving your horse a tree branch or a branch from an edible shrub occasionally to help keep its teeth in working order. Educate yourself about available feeds and use your knowledge to choose wisely for your horse.

In the wild, horses ate very little if any grain except for natural grasses and plants that had gone to seed. Since plant seeds ripen in the fall, the timing was good for the horse since it could gain extra weight to carry

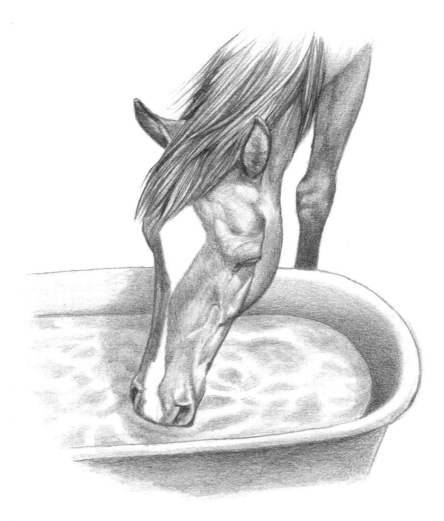

Fresh water

Horses prefer drinking water out of a trough or bucket. Cool, clean water should always be available.

it through the winter months. If your horse has a moderate to heavy workload, grain may be an important component of his diet. Modern, domesticated horses are often fed too much grain considering their workload and body condition. This leads not only to obesity, but also to additional health problems.

Wild horses foraged for feed on the ground for the most part, occasionally reaching up for tree branches or into bushes and chewing on coarser vegetation. Most feeders in barns and stalls force a horse to eat with the neck extended and the head raised instead of lowered. With the neck extended and the head up, the horse cannot properly chew its feed, the amount of saliva decreases, tooth wear is uneven and the possibility of choke or obstruction increases. In addition, fine debris and grass particles bombard the horse's face and neck and can lead to respiratory problems as the horse inhales the falling dust and debris. Use a feeder when feeding your horse. It doesn't have to be fancy, but should keep the horse from eating directly off the ground and ingesting sand or other indigestible matter that might cause colic or poor absorption of feed. As an alternative to using a feeder, you can also feed on stall mats to reduce the amount of sand ingested.

In his natural environment, a horse is a forager, not a grazer. The difference is that a grazer has evolved or been bred for high quality pasture and simply eats, whereas a forager has evolved in variable quality grassland so they spend much of their time looking for the most juicy and nutritious plants and avoiding noxious or unhealthy plants.

A horse's digestive system is both complex and sensitive. With a relatively small stomach, a horse needs to eat small amounts often and the feed needs to contain a high percentage of fibrous material to ensure safe passage through the complex digestive system. Most horse nutritionists recommend splitting the horse's feed into at least two or more feedings each day, usually first thing in the morning and then again in the late afternoon or early evening depending on your schedule.

Foraging activity also provides mental concentration and stimulation for a horse that is more or less confined for much of his day. Since the modern way of feeding horses greatly reduces both the time and the mental challenge associated with food, horse owners need to be creative in reproducing methods of feeding as closely related to the natural way a horse forages as possible.

Your horse should also be provided with a salt mineral block that can be licked to obtain salt and other minerals needed for health and well being. In addition to basic feed your horse will enjoy treats such as pieces of apple and carrots cut small enough to prevent choking and providing these treats gives you another positive way to interact with your horse.

Check your horse's water supply at least twice a day -- morning and evening. Horses should have a continual plentiful supply of fresh, clean water for drinking. The average horse drinks 8 to 10 gallons a day with minimum exercise.

Exercise and physical conditioning

Making sure that your horse gets at least thirty minutes of exercise is a paramount factor when it comes to horse health and well being. This can be riding, lunging, or walking, but should be of sufficient duration and intensity to give the horse a good work out. Without sufficient exercise horses tend to store pent-up energy and become less manageable as time goes on. Some horses turn to stereotypies such as stall walking when they don't have sufficient exercise.

Physical activity is crucial to a horse's well-being. Horses have 216 individual bones held together by ligaments and surrounded by muscles. Because the horse is such an athletic animal, keeping those bones, ligaments and muscles toned and in good working order through exercise builds stamina, endurance and resistance to disease. Lucky is the horse that has a large pasture in which to run and play

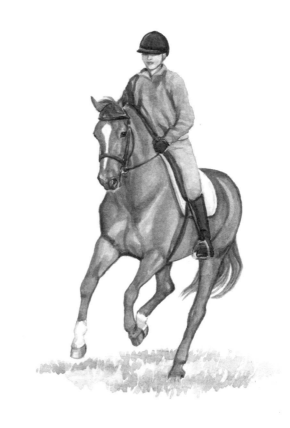

Equine fitness explained

For most horse owners, riding is the principal reason for owning a horse. Avoid injury to your horse by learning the fundamentals of equine conditioning. Learn about it in Chapter 4.

and graze for much of the day. Unfortunately most horses don't have this luxury, and even when they do, they need some supervision, especially if other horses are in the pasture to make sure they don't become injured.

Daily exercise facilitates bone strength and development, improves the functioning of the heart, increases tendon and ligament strength an aids motility of the digestive tract, as well as increasing secretions in the lungs. At low levels, exercise improves the immune system and essentially keeps the horse's body in good working order.

Young horses are especially at risk if they are stabled most of the time. Orthopedic disease and malformations of the limbs, bones, joints and feet because of a lack of exercise lead to lameness and other problems that affect the soundness of the horse. In addition, the horse's mental state is affected and behavioral problems related to pent-up energy and associated with confinement develop. When you do try to ride or exercise the horse, it may respond by bucking or kicking. Cribbing, stall walking, weaving, wind sucking and other vices or stereotypies may become part of the horse's personality due to confinement and lack of exercise.

> ## Note
> ### Hiring an exercise rider
> Be aware of liability issues, but hiring a responsible 4-H, pony club, or collegiate equestrian to ride your horses during the week is an excellent way of keeping your horses in better shape.

For most horses, riding is the best exercise. If the horse is pastured and free to move about, it will need less work-out time. Like humans, horses like a varied exercise routine, so vary the route for your rides and trot up and down hills or over varied, but safe terrain when possible. Once your horse is accustomed to daily physical activity, you can up the pace with riding at a trot and cantering for longer distances. Gradually increase both the length of the exercise and the amount of work required of the horse. Trainers estimate that it takes eight to ten weeks of regular exercise for one to two hours a day to get your horse reasonably fit.

If at all possible, allow your horse free exercise time in a pasture or paddock. Horses can work out the kinks when they have enough room to run, stop, turn, kick up the heels and just be horses. If you cannot exercise your horse on a daily basis, you might want to hire someone who can exercise the horse for you. Be sure that the person is fully acquainted with the horse and with the exercise program you want carried out.

Another way to provide exercise for horses is with a hot or mechanical walker which is an automatic device built like a merry-go-round that the horse can be hooked up to for exercise. Many boarding stables have hot walkers, so if your horse is being boarded you can ask them to hook your horse up to it on the days you can't exercise it. If you can afford a hot walker of your own, you can be doing other things while the horse is being exercised. Just make sure you are alert in case the horse tires too much or something goes wrong with the walker.

Exercise is not only good for the horse's physical health but also a good source of mental stimulation. This is true for both natural exercise such as running about in a pasture and training exercise such as round pen work, lunging and riding. The benefit of exercise in preventing and reducing the development of boredom-related behavioral problems such as wood chewing is noted in a study by the Illinois Movement keeps the horse's circulation working properly, both blood circulation and lymphatic fluid circulation. Every step a horse takes helps to keep their circulation working by 'pumping' fluid back up the legs. The hoof of the horse has evolved to expand to absorb the downward pressure of the horse as the hoof touches the ground and contract to help push fluid upwards again as the hoof leaves the ground. Horses that do not move enough tend to develop problems in the lower legs which tend to fill with fluid when the horse stands still for too long. This fluid build up usually disappears once the horse is exercised.

Horses provided access to paddocks or pasture benefit from opportunities to exercise, with activity positively associated with paddock size. Given room to run and engage in playful activities with other horses helps keep horses physically and mentally fit. Horses appear to be motivated to perform exercise in its own right, with motivation building up and compensatory activity performed after periods of deprivation. Furthermore, horses provided with turn-out display more varied rolling behavior, which is believed to be associated with comfort. In a study of racing horses, benefits of regular turn-out also included less aggression directed toward handlers.

Irregular exercise predisposes horses to "tying up" also known as exertional myopathy with azoturia being the more severe form. It is also known as "Monday morning disease" because it often occurs when a horse has rested, been fed a working ration, and not had sufficient exercise over

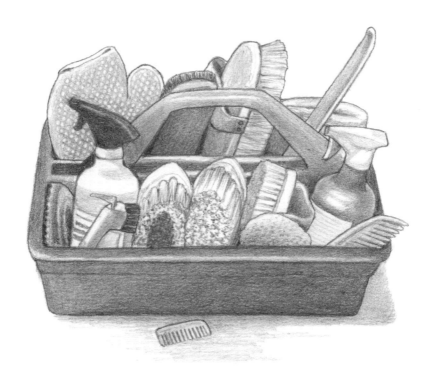

A good scratch on the back

Most horses love being groomed. The grooming activity is one that can create a stronger bond between you and your horse. Grooming also helps you note your horse's physical condition and possible injuries.

a weekend. The horse is then stiff and sore when returning to activity on Monday morning.

Most horses tend to get either too little or too much exercise. That is because they are dependent on us and cannot make their own determination about when to start and stop. Most trainers and horse experts maintain that a horse's daily exercise or work should be sufficient to cause the horse's pulse, respiration, and perspiration output to increase to the point that they are noticeable. Once that point is reached, the horse has had enough exercise for its physical condition and should be allowed to cool down. An older horse in training is going to need time to warm up, so taking time for walking before going on to more demanding exercise is important. For more information related to exercise see the chapter on Fitness and Conditioning

Grooming, bathing and a daily once-over

While you are grooming or bathing your horse, the time is right to combine the grooming or bathing with a daily once over. Observing a horse for potential problems can help owners find concerns before they become larger problems. Note any injuries to the horse's body and legs. Check for sores or signs of infection and note your horse's energy level. Do you see any signs of distress in the horse? When responsible for a horse, an owner must be very observant. Knowing what is normal and what is not for each individual horse can alert the owner or caretaker to a problem before it becomes a big issue. Anytime a horse deviates from normal behavior it is cause for a closer look. If the horse does not appear to feel well, its vital signs should be taken and possibly the veterinarian contacted.

The simple act of performing a daily once-over takes only minutes a day but can keep small problems small and help prevent problems from becoming life threatening thereby saving you vet bills, time and anxiety about your horse's health.

When it comes to grooming or bathing your horse, books, blogs, and many magazine articles have been written about the tools and equipment needed by horse owners to keep their horses well-groomed and clean. Minimalists go with the very basics, but other horse owners fill their barns and tack rooms with all kinds of tools, some of which they never use. Keeping your horse well-groomed is important not only for appearance, but also for your horse's health. Having a good basic knowledge about how to care for your horse's skin and coat and the best products available will enable you to recognize skin or coat conditions that need attention as you proceed with your daily grooming of your horse.

The grooming supplies that you choose for your horse's care should work well for you and be organized to save time and effort as you care for your horse on a daily basis. The basic grooming supplies you will need include a curry comb, stiff and soft brushes, a soft cloth, mane and tail brush, shedding blade, hoof pick, and a hoof brush. You will also want to include shampoo, conditioner and bathing supplies depending on the activity level of your horse and the environmental conditions where it lives. Some horses can go for weeks and months without being bathed, others, including show horses, will need more frequent bathing and grooming to keep them in tip-top showing condition.

Before you start the grooming process you should have your horse tied securely or cross-tied. When a horse is loose you may not have the control that you need, and every horse needs to learn to stand still at grooming time, so this is a good training lesson as well.

Facing the rear, pick a side to start on (I suggest varying that side all of the time, repetitive habits become training) and start with the feet. Pick all four feet, going heel to toe, clean out the hoof and make sure it is free of all debris.

- Starting with your curry comb and the top of the neck, work in light circles and begin the process of cleaning their skin of all mud and debris. You may not need this step if they are not hairy or muddy. Work your way down the body all the way to the tail region, being careful of sensitive skin areas.
- Follow this with the body brush and don't forget to clean their head the horse's head.
- Cleaning the horse's face and nostrils with a damp cloth. Check the interior of the ears as well.
- Next comes the mane and tail. Brush to remove dirt and debris. After this is done, you may want to use a detangle spray. Work your way through any tangles you find.
- Clean the horse's sheath and tail area and if your horse is a mare clean the udders and under the tail area, since these area get the loose, pill-like dirt buildup that creates an itch for the horse.

When grooming your horse, follow five simple safety rules to keep the experience productive and pleasurable and enhance your relationship with your horse.

- Never groom a horse that is loose. Always make sure the horse is properly secured before you begin.
- Never stand directly in front or behind your horse when grooming. Stand off to the side of the legs, in case the horse kicks or begins moving.
- Never sit or kneel down while working on the horse's legs or lower part of the body. Crouch, squat, or bend over and be pre-

pared to move quickly if the horse moves or strikes out.

- Never duck under the horse's belly. The surprise factor may literally "kick" in.
- Never expect a new horse to welcome grooming activities. Use caution and get to know the horse before attempting to brush the underbelly or detangle the tail, for example.

Daily grooming is not only important for your horse's appearance but also for the health benefits of maintaining healthy skin, coat and hoofs. Along with the absolute essentials of feeding, watering and exercising, daily grooming pays dividends in many ways for both you and your horse.

Bathing a horse is a big chore, so make sure

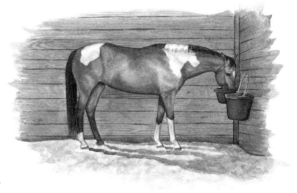

Horse housing explained

Horses have minimal need for housing in most circumstances, but a barn or shelter structure will make your life much easier. Learn about healthy barn living in Chapter 6

you have the time to do it before getting started. At a minimum it will take 20 to 30 minutes to thoroughly wash and rise the horse, plus another 30 to 45 minutes to thoroughly dry it. If you have access to a wash rack, use the hitches for tying the horse. If you are not sure how your horse will respond to being bathed, have someone help you get started and observe carefully how the horse reacts to the procedures. If the horse appears to panic, either hold off giving the bath or take your time and have someone there to help you. Depending on your horse, you may want to use cross ties or tie the horse securely to a hitching post.

You may want to use a garden hose for your water supply, but during cold weather you will need approximately 72 gallons of lukewarm water on hand. You can purchase an electrical bucket warmer at feed and tack stores with which to heat your water supply. Wear shoes and clothes that you don't mind getting wet, but never bathe your horse while going barefoot for obvious reasons. Assemble your supplies including shampoo, conditioner, body sponge, face sponge, a sweat scraper and a supply of drying towels along with a cooler or sweat sheet to protect the horse during cold weather.

Beginning on the front left side of the horse, run lukewarm water from a garden hose, or use lukewarm water from a bucket to wet down the legs to get the horse used to the water and let it know it is going to be bathed. After the horse adjusts to the water, proceed to move the hose up to where the neck joins the head and wet the body all the way to the rear end. If using a bucket of lukewarm water, apply water with a soaked sponge. Apply shampoo to the sponge and lather the horse's coat starting at the neck and working down across the body. Scrub underneath the horse and along the back to remove any encrusted sweat and dirt that has accumulated. Wash the horse's legs and the outsides of its hoofs. Once you have loosened the dirt and sweat, use the hose or water from the bucket and rinse the shampoo from your horse's coat. Be sure to rinse thoroughly since any soap or shampoo residue may irritate the horse's skin. Use the same procedure on the other side of the horse. Then shampoo, condition and rinse the horse's mane. Wash the horse's tail using enough lather to penetrate all the hair. Rinse and condition the tail and then rinse again making sure that all residue is thoroughly removed. Wash the horse's head. Some horse's do not like having their heads and faces washed so be gentle and considerate using lukewarm water from a bucket. Often shampoo is not needed on the head and face, and warm water will suffice to clean the facial areas and ears. Don't squirt the horse in the face with a hose. Most horses will object and this can lead to complications the next time you want to bathe your horse.

Note
Wash and roll

After a wonderful cleansing bath, the first thing your horse will want to do is roll in the dirt. This isn't necessarily bad as rolling in the speeds drying and is fun to watch. However, if you need to keep your horse clean, put them in a bedded stall after washing. Another tip - spray your horse with a silicone based spray, such as ShowSheen®, after washing. When the coat dries, removal of dust and dirt is accomplished with a quick brush or moistened towel.

Depending on your horse, you will want to bathe the private parts of the horse on a regular basis. With some geldings, it's better to let your vet clean the sheath because a sedative may be needed before the gelding will allow the cleaning to take place. With mares, the cleaning job is relatively easy. Wearing latex gloves, clean out the waxy substance that builds up between the teats and between her back legs. Wet the areas with warm water and apply shampoo. Rinse thoroughly to remove all soap. Be cautious because the mare may not like the process and may attempt to kick you.

After the bath, whisk away as much water as possible by using a sweat scraper. Dry the horse's face with a towel being careful to not frighten it by letting it sniff the towel before you touch it to the face. If it is a sunny or warm day, walk your horse preferably on a hard surface or on grass to avoid any dust or dirt getting on his freshly washed feet and legs. If the day is cool, dry the horse as well as possible using towels and cover it with a sheet that will absorb any dampness. Depending on the temperature, you may want to blanket the horse.

Never put a wet horse back in its stall, paddock or pasture. Doing so is not healthy for the horse, especially if it is cold enough that it will be chilled. Also, the horse may decide to get down and roll and most of your hard work will come to naught.

Shelter and a quiet environment

Many factors need to be considered when it comes to housing your horse. Some people prefer to board their horse either at an established stable or on a local farm. Others prefer to have their horses on their property and to build barns for housing the animals, equipment and feed. The choice is often dictated by the circumstances of the horse owner. Obviously, having a property that is suitable (and legal) for horse housing is not always a choice.

Time is also a big consideration. Feeding and cleaning stalls takes time that not every horse owner is willing to spend. Also, many peopled enjoy the camaraderie that they experience at "the barn." For these owners, stabling at a barn is preferred. Others enjoy the daily activity of taking care of their horse or horses. They like being able to casually visiting with their horses on the spur of the moment. There are other advantages to having your horse close by for routine riding and exercise activities.

In making decisions regarding housing for your horse, you will need to make sure you consider the horse's needs, what you intend to do with your horse, and how much you can afford to spend on housing your horse. Basically, horses need shelter from uncomfortable weather conditions whether it be heat, cold, wind or snow and a safe, dry place to eat. For ages, horses have survived very well in most climates with relatively modest shelters. If your horse is strictly for pleasure riding during good weather, again, a modest shelter with space for exercise, some pasture access, and a dry place for feeding may meet the horse's needs. On the other hand, if your horse is to participate in shows, competitions or races, you will need to consider more protection from weather and a more elaborate facility along with more sophisticated trailer and travel considerations.

The local weather conditions in your area will determine how elaborate your shelter for your horse needs to be. In a temperate climate, a three-sided shelter or a cold barn to provide protection from weather and wind and a dry place to feed the horse may be sufficient along with a dry storage area for hay, tack, and other necessary equipment. In colder climates or in cases of competition horses with demanding schedules, more elaborate structures including barns, stalls, arenas and exercise paddocks may be necessary.

Meeting the needs of your particular horse

The temperament of the horse including the need for sociability is an important consideration. A few horses seem to be fairly contented in more or less isolated conditions, while others tend to develop stereotypies when left without the company of other horses and humans.

If your horse is a show or competitive animal, your decisions regarding housing should include the special requirements necessary to allow for the exercise, grooming, and trailering of the horse.

Effectively housing and managing a horse, takes a great deal of planning, time, and money. The more research and fact-finding you can do in preparation for owning and housing a horse, the better your chances for a healthy and happy experience for all concerned. The size and location of stalls is an important consideration and should be determined with the horse's size and freedom of movement in mind. Consideration of existing or future pastures and paddocks need to be part of planning for maximum usefulness of any additions to the site along with the number of horses that will be using the facilities. Driveways and access for trailers and other equipment should be high on the priority list both for convenience and safety.

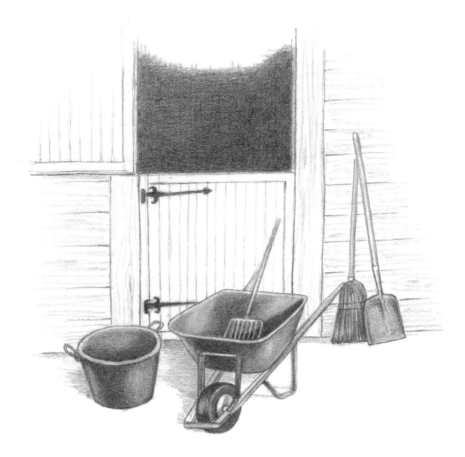

Safe and clean

Keeping your barnyard clean and tidy results in better health for your horse and better safety for you. Get quality implements and have a proper location for keeping them.

Horses need to spend as much time as possible outside and have a large area for free exercise for maximum well being. Adequate space provides more opportunities for mental stimulation simply through movement. A large stall is better than a small one, as are a large paddock and a large pasture. The importance of the horse's housing is proportional to the amount of time the horse spends inside; a horse that spends much of its time in a stall deserves a large one whereas a horse which has free access to pasture and only enters its stall to sleep or for occasional shelter has

143

less need of the larger space.

Horses require a quiet environment for maximum well-being. As prey animals, barking dogs, honking horns, sudden bursts of loud laughter or unexplained sounds cause the horse's nervous system to go into over-drive. This can be damaging to both the horse's physical and emotional health if it is a daily occurrence.

> ## Note
> ### Non-equine horse companions?
>
> For many horse owners, cost or space may limit the ability to have more than one horses. Fortunately, horses readily accept companionship from smaller equines, or even non-equines. Consider a donkey, goat or sheep as a suitable companion for your horse.

In addition, a horse's sight often keeps the horse on alert. Horses do not see the world as we do. They have what is known as monocular vision as well as binocular vision. With the monocular vision, they are able to see to each side of their head much better than humans and are constantly aware of what is going on around them. They also have binocular vision, which allows them to see objects in front of them. However, horses are unable to see approximately 4 feet directly in front of them which can lead to unexpected surprises that impact their environment.

Horses also hear much better than humans. All of these factors can be possible explanations of why they seem to spook easily and without warning on occasion especially when their environment contains abrupt surprises especially noises. When a horse is stressed, he may also show signs of agitation. A horse that is agitated may lay his ears back and swish his tail. Noise is a recognized stressor in horses.

Socialization and companionship

Horses are herd animals and as such are most comfortable when part of a herd. Most horses needs at least one other companion animal to help relieve stress and provide a social context. Periodic human company is no substitute for this. In some cases, they will accept other animals such as goats or sheep as companion animals. As prey species, horses are highly motivated to interact with individuals of their own species for comfort, play, access to food and shelter resources, and as an anti-predator strategy. During fearful situations and when separated from closely bonded companions, restlessness, pacing, and vocalizations occur and suggest experiences of acute anxiety and distress. Confining horses for long periods may produce behavioral problems including depression or aggression that sometimes progresses to exhibition of stereotypies, commonly referred to as vices.

Horses housed singly display greater activity and reduced foraging compared with horses kept in pairs or groups. Horses housed singly also display more aggression toward human handlers and learn new tasks more slowly than horses housed in groups.

In additional to the mental benefits, group animals tend to be much more physically active than solitary ones, which has physical health benefits. With modern domesticated horses, the design of the stables can allow for social interaction among horses and other animals. For example, stall walls which are low enough that the horses can see each other and even touch noses allow for a level of companionship, as do stall doors that allow the horses to stick their heads out and see each other. For more information about horses and their needs read the Behavior chapter.

General care supplies for maintaining horse health

One of the most essential tools you need to care for your horse is a well-stocked first aid kit with wound dressings, antiseptic solution, bandages, scissors, surgical and duct tape, leg wraps, ointment, tweezers, Q-tips, spray bottles, towels for applying pressure to slow or stop bleeding, a clean bucket, and your veterinarians phone number for use in case of emergency.

A weight tape comes in handy when you want to quickly estimate your horse's weight. Weight tapes are available at feed and tack stores. If a commercial weight tape isn't available, you can use an ordinary measuring tape and consult a horse's weight table following the directions given in the table.

Many horse owners find a heart monitor to be a necessity to help keep track of what is going on with their horse's heart during different activities and as a key component for measuring the health of the horse. A variety of commercial heart monitors are available to measure fitness, well being and sports performance. Although not absolutely necessary, they help keep track of a horse's fitness. Heart monitors are accurate, reliable and easy to use during rest, exercise, and recovery.

Every responsible horse owner needs to be able to check a horse's vital signs at a moment's notice. Supplies you will need include a rectal thermometer (digital or bulb), for taking temperature; K-Y Jelly or other water=based jelly for easy insertion; a stethoscope, although not absolutely necessary a stethoscope can come in handy when checking a horse's pulse, respiration rate, and also for checking for gut sounds in cases of colic and other conditions.

Medications

Some basic medications are often necessary for good horse health and it pays to have a supply of these medications readily available. Common oral medications that you may want to keep on hand include anti-inflammatories and antibiotics, along with NSAIDs and other commonly prescribed drugs and treatments. As you become more experienced, and gain the trust of your veterinarian, he may prescribe some common medications for you to stock in your medicine cabinet.

If your horse needs daily injections or medications, your veterinarian can show you how to do the injections or how to get the horse to swallow oral medications. Always listen to and follow your veterinarians advice when using medications or prescriptions and check expiration dates regularly to make sure they are still viable.

Your horse's vital signs

A horse's main vital signs include heart or pulse rate, body temperature, respiration or frequency of breathing and gut sounds.

These vital signs should be observed at rest on a number of occasions, to determine normal levels for each individual horse. Heart and breathing rates vary depending on the age and fitness of the individual, being higher in foals and old horses, and in those that are unfit.

Changes to the normal vital signs, observed at rest, are often key indicators of pain or illness. Normal ranges at rest are as follows:

Vital Sign	Normal range
Heart rate	28 - 40 beats per minute (bpm)
Temperature	99 - 101.5° F (37 - 38° C)
Respiration	12 - 20 breaths per minute
Gut sounds	Bubbling or gurgling 6 - 12 times per minute.

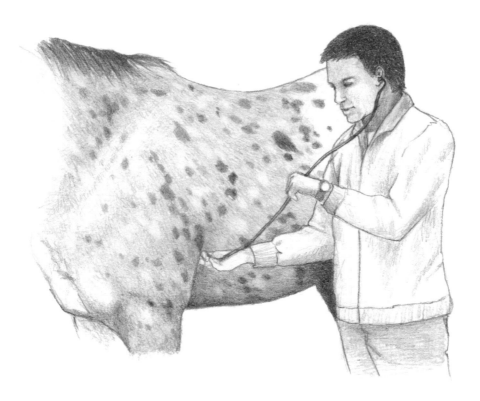

Measuring heart rate

One of the more difficult vital signs to obtain, even using a stethescope, it takes practice and care to measure your horse's pulse rate. Ask your veterinarian to show you how.

Virtually all vital signs naturally increase significantly during exercise and gradually return to normal as the horse recovers – the fitter the horse, the quicker rates will return to normal.

Heart rate

Exercise, physical condition, environmental temperature, disease, excitement, and age can influence a horse's heart rate.

Pulse rates of more than 80 bpm, in the absence of excitement or exercise, may indicate heat stroke, severe dehydration, colic, shock, infection, advanced heart and lung diseases, or septicemia. Call your veterinarian!

A pulse rate under 20 bpm suggests low body temperature, heart disease,

147

pressure on the brain, or a possible preterminal state with an impending collapse of circulation.

Taking a horse's pulse can be very difficult, even for an experienced veterinarian. The horse pulse is rather slow, and finding just the right spot to feel the pulse, especially on a moving animal, will test your patience, but since the horse's heart rate is important under many circumstance, it is vitally important for a horse owner to be able to take the horse's pulse.

The pulse, which reflects the heart rate, can be taken at any point where a large artery is located just beneath the skin.

Three points to locate and use to take the horse's pulse are:
- The external maxillary artery that crosses the lower border of the jawbone
- The radial artery at the back inside of the knee
- The digital artery, located below the fetlock at the inside of the ankle

Sounds easy doesn't it? Actually, finding and determining a horse's pulse can be difficult, even for professionals. It takes just the right touch and plenty of practice. Fortunately, most people can learn to use a stethoscope to hear the heart beat with practice.

How to take your horse's heart rate

To find your horse's pulse on the maxillary artery, stand slightly to the side of the horse's head and cup your hand with your first two fingers along the inside of the jawbone, just below the heavy muscles of the cheek. Feel along the inside of the jawbone until you consistently feel the pulse beat. Looking at your watch, count the beats for 30 seconds, then double the count to give you bpm.

If you choose to take the pulse at the inside back of the knee on the radial artery crouch facing the limb, then place your hand around the back of the knee with the pads of your fingers pressing on the radial artery. Taking the pulse here is similar to taking your pulse at the wrist. Once your fingers locate the strong, consistent pulse beat, count the beats for 30 seconds and double the count for the bpm.

If you choose to take the pulse below the fetlock at the inside of the ankle, crouch facing the limb and locate the digital artery with the pads of your fingers. The pulse may be best found on the inside or outside branch of the digital artery. Place the pads of your fingers on the artery and count the beats for 30 seconds, then double for bpm.

A simpler method to get your horse's heart rate is to listen with a stethoscope. For most people, including most veterinarians, this is the preferred method. You can purchase a quality stethoscope for under $100. Our favorite is the Littmann Classic, used by medical professionals.

If you choose to use a stethoscope to listen for your horse's heart rate, properly place the stethoscope ear tips in your ears. Note that the ear tips should be pointing forward for the proper and comfortable placement.

Position yourself on the left side (mounting side) of the horse, at the front shoulder, facing to the rear of the animal.

Locate the elbow of the horse and place the diaphragm just behind the elbow on the chest wall. Press moderately and listen for a low dub-dub sound. When you can clearly hear the sound, count each dub-dub for 30 seconds, then double for the bpm.

Your horse's pulse should be strong, steady, and regular. Knowing your horse's regular pulse rate is helpful in determining the state of your horse's health in cases of illness or injury.

Temperature

A horse's temperature is another important vital sign that helps both horse owners and veterinarians determine the state of a horse's health.

According to AAEP guidelines, in an adult horse, any body temperature at or below 101.5° F is considered normal. Individual horse's normal temperatures may vary. In horses that appear healthy otherwise, there's no such thing as a temperature that's too low. Readings above 101.5° F, on the other hand, are cause for concern.

Strenuous exercise can raise your horse's body temperature by a few degrees, but that should return to normal within 90 minutes of finishing the exercise. If it remains elevated for longer than that, he may be dealing with an underlying illness or he may suffer from anhydrosis, a condition in which horses lose the ability to cool themselves by sweating.

Temperature-taking is vital for good equine husbandry, so all horses should learn to stand quietly for the procedure from an early age. It is completely painless, and almost all horses tolerate it easily. However, it can be extremely dangerous for the human handler to attempt doing it with an uncooperative horse, such as a misbehaving yearling. When in doubt, ask one or more experienced horse people to help you get the job done.

How to take your horse's temperature

To measure your horse's temperature, use a plastic or digital "oral" or "rectal" thermometer. Oral and rectal thermometers are essentially the same thing. Digital thermometers are safer (harder to break and mercury-free) than glass ones, and so much faster that you don't need to resort to the old, occasionally unreliable method of clipping the thermometer to the horse's tail while you wait for the temperature to register. The least expensive models read in about 30 seconds, whereas slightly more expensive models read within 10 seconds.

Take a baseline reading at a time when your horse is relaxed, such as during a meal. If he is young, does not stand tied or you don't know him well, ask a friend to hold him while you take his temperature. If you are on your own, tie him up.

Stand next to your horse's hind leg, facing the direction of his tail, close enough for your shoulder or side to be in contact with him so you'll sense any motion in his body if he begins to get antsy. If you are right-handed, stand on his left side, with the thermometer in your right hand; if you're left-handed, stand on his right side, with the thermometer in your left hand. Throughout the procedure, be careful not to turn your body to face his leg, as this puts you in a very vulnerable position because your knees won't be free to bend if he kicks or moves suddenly in your direction.

Next, place your arm closest to the horse across his croup and gently grasp the top of his tail in your hand. Raise it up high enough to give your other hand access to the anus. If your horse is young or you're not sure how he reacts to thermometers, gently touch the skin around the outside of the anus with the thermometer before inserting it. This will help to accustom him to the feel of it. Then guide the end of the thermometer into the rectum, pressing it several inches inside, leaving the digital screen outside the body so you can see it while it registers the temperature.

Continue holding the tail and the end of the thermometer firmly until the final reading is clear (consult the manual that comes with the thermometer ahead of time to see exactly how your particular brand indicates this). Then gently remove the thermometer and double-check the reading.

Use this baseline temperature for comparison when your horse shows signs of stress or illness. If his temperature goes above normal, consult your veterinarian.

Respiration rate

Another indication of your horse's health is the respiration rate: The average respiration rate of an adult horse at rest is 8-15 breaths per minute. A horse's respiration rate increases with hot or humid weather, exercise, fever or pain. Rapid breathing at rest should receive veterinary attention, and keep in mind that the respiration rate should never exceed the pulse rate. A horse should also spend equal time inhaling and exhaling.

How to take your horse's respiration rate

To take the respiration rate, watch or feel your horse's rib cage/belly for one minute. Be sure to count 1 inhale and 1 exhale as one breath (not as two). Each breath is fairly slow. If you are having difficulty seeing the rib cage move, try watching the horse's nostrils or place your hand in front of the nostrils to feel the horse exhale.

An even better method is to place a stethoscope to the horse's windpipe to listen to his breathing. This will also give you strange sounds if the horse's windpipe is blocked by mucous or if the he has allergies or heaves.

Gut sounds

Known as "Borborygmus" the gut sounds of a horse digesting his feed are often important in determining the state of the horse's health. The absence of gut sounds is more indicative of a problem than excessive gut sounds. Usually, an absence of gut sounds indicates colic.

How to listen to your horse's gut sounds

To hear your horse's gut sounds, press your ear up against your horse's barrel just behind his last rib. If you hear gurgling noises, he's fine. Be sure to check gut sounds from both sides. If you do not hear any sounds, try using a stethoscope in the same area.

You should be able to hear normal gurgling sounds on both sides of the horse's abdomen near the flanks. Usually two long rolls, followed by several small gurgles will be heard over a period of about one minute. Gut sounds should always be present. If you don't hear any sounds or if there is a consistent, fast gurgling instead of the natural combination of rolls and gurgles, contact your veterinarian.

Other health parameters to note

1. Capillary refill: This is an indication of blood circulation. Normal refill time is 1 to 2 seconds.
2. Mucous membranes: The mucous membranes line the horse's eyelids, gums and nostrils, and the color is another indicator of blood circulation. A healthy horse's mucous membranes are moist and pink.
3. Dehydration: Healthy horses drink a minimum of 7 gallons of

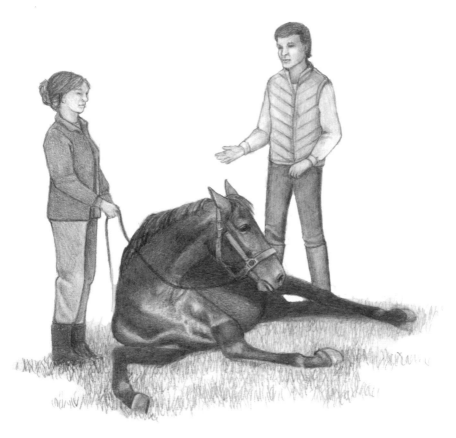

A sad moment

Thankfully, horses live a long time, and can be enjoyed for 30 years or more. However, when the time comes, making the decision to euthanize is never easy.

water a day and average around 10 to 12 gallons a day with a performance horse requiring up to 24 gallons per day depending on heat, humidity and workload.

4. General demeanor: Over time you will learn to read your horse's health by observing the look in his eye and the way that he acts or reacts to you. If your horse seems off, it is wise to check his vital signs for signals of disease.

What is "normal" can vary greatly between individual animals and conditions. Get to know your horse's vital signs by checking them occasionally. Also, it is a good practice to check the vital signs and be ready to discuss them when you call the vet for a problem.

Euthanasia

Anyone who owns horses will eventually face the mind-numbing task of deciding when, how, and where to end the life of a horse.

In the worst-case scenario, due to a sudden, severe injury or the onslaught of severe transmittable disease, an owner may have to make a quick decision regarding whether to spend huge sums of money without knowing the potential outcome, or working with a veterinarian to euthanize the horse in a humane manner.

By thinking ahead and doing some planning for the inevitable, a horse owner will be able to make rational decisions and have time to share the plan with others who may become involved if the owner is not on the scene when the final decisions have to be made. In any case, this is a task that demonstrates ultimate respect for the horse.

No one wants a horse to go through undue suffering because of illness or chronic lameness or the debilitation that comes because of age or progressive disease. Veterinarians often advise horse owners to consider euthanasia when a horse is suffering with inoperable colic or other serious health conditions.

When foals are born with genetic or other serious defects that would keep them from having any quality of life, rather than have them suffer, again euthanasia needs to be considered.

National, state and local ordinances often require euthanasia of a horse that contracts a severe transmittable disease that can spread to other horses.

Behavioral traits that endanger people, other animals, or the horse itself sometimes necessitate euthanasia. This is indeed one of the saddest situations as the decision to put down an otherwise healthy animal is always extremely difficult.

In each case, the right choice is the one that is in the best interest of the horse and the people who care for the animal.

Having a veterinarian involved in making the decision is important, especially if the veterinarian has a history with the horse and knows how it will respond to treatment or other compounding factors, such as the amount of pain involved as a result of injury or illness.

Prepare for what may occur and what will occur

One of the responsibilities of horse ownership is making advance preparations, both for what may occur and what will occur. The death of a horse, whether from natural causes or euthanasia, should be addressed and planned-for so everyone involved with the horse knows what to do when the time comes. Compiling a list of the steps to take and posting it in a convenient place will save stress and time. The list should include the following:

- Phone number of veterinarian, with an alternate to be used in an emergency along with the name and phone number of nearest horse trauma center or hospital
- A written emergency euthanasia plan with acceptable methods to be used as a guideline for humane euthanasia of animals on the premises.
- If the horse is insured, the name and phone number of the insurance company, along with access to a copy of the policy with important guidelines of the policy highlighted. (Note that in many cases, an insurance company will want a second opinion before an insured horse is euthanized.)
- A copy of any local, state, and federal regulations relative to disposal or burial of horses and information about burial sites, rendering services, professional disposal services, and possible sources for cremation of the horse's remains, depending on what best meets the needs and desires of the owner
- The names and phone numbers of reliable backhoe operators that can be called to move the horse's body to a burial site or the phone numbers of removal services. (Your veterinarian probably knows about resources available in the area and may have recommendations for you.)

The decision to euthanize a horse may be made in an emergency on the racetrack, at the scene of an accident, in the corral, or on the trail. Some accidents do not allow any leeway as to when and where because the horse's condition and degree of suffering do not permit transport to a convenient or special facility.

If the decision to euthanize a horse is the result of a chronic progressive illness, debilitation because of age, dangerous behavioral traits, or because the caring of a sick or incapacitated horse is too much of a financial burden, the timing and place of the euthanasia is under the control of the owner and the veterinarian.

A veterinarian can provide medical information and the horse's prognosis along with options, comfort, and support, but the horse's owner has the responsibility for determining that it is time to euthanize the horse. In the past, many veterinarians preferred not to have the owner and family members present during euthanasia because complications may occur that are unpleasant, dangerous, or distressing to those who have had a relationship with the horse.

"Currently euthanasia is being viewed more frequently by veterinary professionals and animal owners alike as both a privilege and a gift that can be lovingly bestowed on ill or injured animals. With this in mind, concerned veterinarians, animal health technicians, and grief counselors from across the country have worked together during the last decade to create and perfect euthanasia protocols that have both the patient's and the client's comfort and well-being in mind."

In the ideal scenario, most veterinarians choose to administer an intravenous barbiturate overdose in a setting familiar to the horse. When the drug is given, the horse loses consciousness and experiences relief from pain almost immediately, breathing stops, and then the heart ceases to beat. This method is very similar to the process people undergo when administered general anesthesia and is accomplished without panic, pain, or trauma.

Confirmation of death may be through the absence of breathing, heartbeat, or a corneal reflex, as tested by the veterinarian. In any case, planning ahead and knowing what to do can be a source of comfort to all involved during this most difficult time.

> Somewhere in time's Own Space
> There must be some sweet pastured place
> Where creeks sing on and tall trees grow
> Some Paradise where horses go,
> For by the love that guides my pen
> I know great horses live again
> ~Stanley Harrison

Conclusion

General care activities are easy to do, not too expensive and are the best insurance against expensive veterinarian bills. All horse owners should learn how to administer oral wormers. Most horse owners will also want to administer routine vaccinations. This is a skill that is easy to learn, and will save you the cost of a veterinarian visit.

Grooming and bathing your horse are activities that will help you bond with your horse, and also establish yourself as a familiar and friendly leader. This chapter taught you the basics of grooming as a part of horse healthcare. A daily once-over will allow you to find and treat small injuries before they become more serious.

A horses vital signs are the starting point of any physical exam. Learning to take your horse's vital signs for your veterinarian will jump-start the diagnostic process, even before the veterinarian arrives.

Nutrition, hoof care and dental care are also routine concerns as part of general care. These topics are covered in-depth within their chapters in this book.

Owning a horse is a big responsibility, and is much more expensive and labor intensive than non-horse owners would imagine. Knowing the basics of general care will help minimize the costs and increase the joy of horse ownership. Indeed, for many horse owners, including the authors of this book, taking care of our horse's health is very satisfying and rewarding. You can take pride in your horse's health, and will be amazed at how nice your horse looks and performs when they are in great health.

Top-5 takeaways
1. Every horse should be on a vaccination and worming schedule. Local area conditions must be considered, so rely on your veterinarian to advise you on what and when you should vaccinate and worm.
2. A daily once-over is the best thing you can do to maintain your horse's health. Demeanor, body condition, heat in legs or feet, attitude are all signals of general health. A good grooming session is called for at least weekly.
3. A horse's vital signs can indicate problems with your horse's health. Increased heart rate may be associated with pain or stress. Increased temperature may be associated with infection or disease. Learning to take your horse's vital signs can also help you communicate essential information to your veterinarian prior to a call.
4. A holistic approach is productive for horse well being. This approach includes attention to housing, nutrition, exercise and social interactions with other horses and caretakers.

5. Developing a good relationship with your veterinarian and farrier pays dividends as you learn to take more responsibility for your horse's health. Do not wait until there is a problem to call on these service providers. Get to know them in advance and you will be rewarded with preventative advice, and great service should an emergency arise.

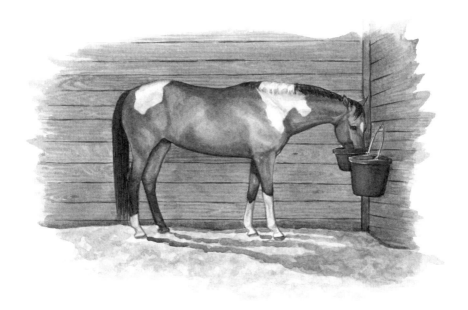

Chapter 6 Healthy Barn

Introduction

The horse barn is a wonderful place. It is active and alive. It is a place to hang-out and to work - two activities that are central to horse ownership. However, aside from being many horse owner's favorite place, barns can also be dangerous.

Horse nature is generally incompatible with confinement in an enclosed space. The horse's number one defense mechanism is reactionary flight. Because of this, care must be taken in the design of any housing structure used for horses to reduce the chance of injury and also to provide for the well-being of the horse.

Fortunately, most horses would prefer to live outside in a never-ending green pasture. For those of you who do not have access to never-ending pasture, this chapter is for you. The number one concern is making your barn a place of safety for both you and your horse. Most of this is common sense, but armed with the information in this chapter, you can take a walk through your barn and probably identify a number of things that should be addressed to increase overall safety.

Beyond safety, our barns must also provide a healthy environment.

Respiratory illnesses, hoof problems, skin conditions - all can result from a barn that is not properly ventilated and maintained properly. Lastly, the mental condition of your horse may be impacted due to poor barn design or a lack of maintenance that results in unsafe conditions.

Is a barn necessary?

Although horses in their natural environment spend their days and nights in the open, they usually seek areas of shelter such as a grove of trees, big boulders, or protective areas next to hills or mountains. To stay healthy, horses need constant access to a dry, safe, comfortable shelter to protect them from rain, wind, and snow. In some areas, a lean-to type shed is sufficient. In other areas, a barn with doors and windows that can be closed during inclement weather is necessary. In warm and sunny weather, the shelter provides your horse with much needed shade and relief from biting insects. In the winter or during cold, rainy, snowy seasons, your horse needs protection from the cold along with protection from wet ground and blustery storms. Having a safe, comfortable place for the horses that you love and care about means that a barn is not just about storing some animals. It's about providing the best that you can for the creatures that mean so much in your life.

At a minimum, you should have a well-constructed, three-sided shed into which your horse can retreat at all times. The entry should have a clear path and the ceilings should be high enough to allow horses to move their heads up and down.

Provisions should be made for natural light and ventilation without being drafty in cold weather. The shelter should be planned so it does not flood during heavy rain or snow melt. Floors should dry quickly, provide good traction for the horse's feet and should be easy to clean since manure will need to be removed on a daily basis.

In addition, most horse owners need an easily accessible place to keep their horse-related tack, grooming supplies, feeding and watering equip-ment, cleaning implements such as shovels, muck rakes, wheelbarrows and the countless other items needed to support a healthy barn. As a horse owner it is important to realize that in most areas, a barn not only adds value to a property, but also saves a horse owner money, time, and effort.

Barn - a pleasant, practical place for horse and human

A well-designed, well-built horse barn is light, airy, pleasant to work in, easy to keep clean-and every bit as comfortable as your home. In the long run, it pays off in lower upkeep costs, fewer vet bills, and added property value.

A healthy barn will be safety-oriented, with exits clearly marked in case of emergency. Ceilings should be 8 to 12 feet high and door frames a minimum of 8 feet high and 4 feet wide for easy ingress and egress. More than one exit should be provided in all cases.

In addition, a barn should protected areas for feed and grain storage that can be rodent proof, thereby saving on the costs of feed. A barn also supplies room for the storage of bedding materials, and other needed horse care supplies close to where they will be used. This saves a horse owner both time and money.

Notables
It's a wonderful "barn" life

If you keep your horse at a commercial stable, you will find that there exists a community of owners that have their horses as a focal point of their social lives. You can learn a lot, and enjoy the hopefully cordial atmosphere, but beware of well intentioned advice. Use your equine healthcare team, namely your veterinarian and farrier, to advise you concerning health related matters. This advice applies to on-line "forums" where well intentioned but bad advice is routinely provided.

A well designed barn will help you save energy and time by having everything needed to care for your horse from water buckets to grooming supplies in a well-organized central location. In addition, the mess that naturally goes along with horses can be minimized when you identify all potential sources of mess and plan your layout to confine that mess. Keeping mucking implements near stalls and grooming supplies near the bathing area will save you countless steps on a daily basis.

A well-organized barn will have a secure place for medications and deworming supplies you use on a regular basis plus a well-supplied first aid emergency kit that allows ready access in case of injury to a horse or a sudden onset illness.

The barn structure

Although most equines prefer to be outdoors, there are occasions when having covered shelter is important. These include periods of extreme weather including lightning and thunder storms, periods of illness or lameness, or when access to turn-out is limited.

Before deciding on the architectural details of your barn, make sure that the chosen site is appropriate and conducive to good horse health. Look for a barn site that's well drained and offers easy connection to utilities and to the road and/ or your driveway. When you find your site, spend time there on a blustery day to identify the prevailing wind direction; then orient your barn with that in mind.

> ## Note
> ### Stall flooring
>
> Most horse owners use the natural soil as the flooring of stalls and breezeways. Depending on soil type, natural drainage occurs, keeping stalls relatively clean and odor free. If your natural soil is sand, take caution because sand ingested with hay can accumulate in the color and lead to colic. In most cases, 4' x 6' rubber stall mats help you keep the stall clean and reduces the chances for sand colic.

You want good air circulation, but you don't want your center aisle to be a wind tunnel. If strong winds come from all four directions, you might build a square barn with entrances on all four sides and the ability to close down any one, two, or three as needed.

Situating a barn well affects working conditions. Experts advise avoiding low-lying areas or those at the bottom of a hill because runoff from rain and snow will be a problem. If wet weather brings flooding and run-off, wet areas around the barn are troublesome to work in and can become breeding grounds for insects that carry diseases. You may think that standing or pooling water near your barn is simply a nuisance, but it may be a bigger issue and can pose a threat to your horse's health and erode the structure of your barn. Build downwind of any residential buildings to minimize the flies and odors. Orient the barn so it takes advantage of winter sun, avoids the hottest summer sun and catches summer winds for ventilation. The location of roads, including service roads, should also be considered.

Function, efficiency and safety

The design of a barn impacts both the time and the money you spend to keep your horse happy and healthy. Whether you're building or redoing a small private setup or a large professional training operation, well-planned storage in your barn can save time and supplies. Since most horses need

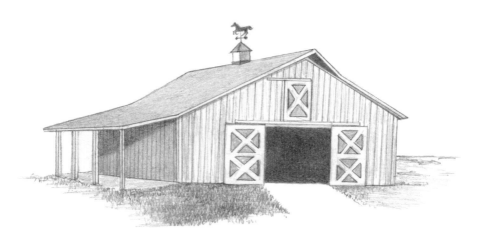

A home for your horse

Many horse owners prefer to keep their animals at their home. Building a barn, or rehabbing an existing barn requires careful planning with attention to both the needs of the horse and safety.

their feedings of hay on a daily basis, the question about where to store hay is important to the over-all design of any barn.

Many safety experts caution horse owners about storing hay in their barns. By creating a storage area that is outside the barn, but opens to the inside, it is possible to have your hay close enough for ease in feeding, but separate enough to prevent it being a fire hazard. While it's quite convenient to store hay in a loft and drop it into the aisle, it is not only a fire hazard but adds to the barn's dust and allergen levels.

Practicality and barn size matter

An important feature of every barn are the stalls where horses are kept when they cannot be in turnout or pastures. Stalls should be sized according to the size of your animals, and also according to the particular usage of the stall. For example, if you own a cold-blood draft breed, you will need rather large stall sizes for all purposes. For a stall to house draft breeds, you should probably plan for 16 feet by 16 feet at a minimum.

If you breed, and own stallions or mares, the stall sizes will need to be larger. Stallions do better with a larger stall to help them cope with the stress of being an isolated breeding animal. Mares need a larger stall for foaling and for housing when with a nursing foal.

If a stall is where your horse lives all the time except for occasional rides, opt for a larger stall. The most common stall is 12 feet square. The horse needs to be able to move around and get up and down comfortably. Partitions between stalls should be at least 8 feet high to prevent a horse from getting a hoof over them, but they don't necessarily have to be solid from top to bottom. Spaces of an inch or so between wooden boards will enhance ventilation, as will a barred or mesh portion on the top. This configuration also has the benefit of allowing horses, which are herd animals, to see their companions--and provides easy observation of the horses by their humans.

Note
Automatic waterer or bucket?

Studies have shown that watering from a bucket is more likely to encourage water consumption versus an automatic waterer. Especially in periods of fluctuating weather when colics often occur, knowing how much your horse is drinking is a clue to forestall a colic.

Horses drink a lot of water, if using a bucket, it is wise to hang two 5-gallon buckets to always maintain fresh water in front of your horse.

Doors that are open on top or an open door with a stall guard or safety gate will increase visibility, light and ventilation. Bars, however, must not be more than 2 to 3 inches apart, and openings in heavy gauge wire mesh should not be more than 2 inches across to prevent a hoof from getting caught in the mesh. Doors should be wide enough for a wheelbarrow to pass in and out, at least 4 feet. Sliding doors are considered by some horse owners to be better than swinging doors.

Making care-taking easy

Easy access to feed buckets is the quickest and most efficient way to feed without opening and closing stall doors. A swing-out panel with a feed tub in the bottom and a hay rack in the top, or two separate swing-outs can expedite the feeding of horses. Both lock open and shut to avoid being tampered with by a bored horse's lips. While swing-out hay racks are easy to fill, some people prefer feeding hay on the ground as it is more natural for the horse and avoids the dust from hay in mangers placed on a wall.

Although many horses prefer a water bucket which makes it easy for you to know how much the horse is drinking, automatic waterers can be installed, and have the advantage of offering fresh water at all times.

In the feed room, wooden bins lined with metal are one way to keep feed safe from rodents. Whether using trash cans or custom-built bins, elevating them off the ground will make scooping easier. For large barns, a storage bin outside with an auger that opens into the feed room for the delivery of grain is convenient.

Consider convenience

The wash stall is a convenience, but always install a drain from which clogs can be removed easily and put a removable strainer in the drain. Position the hose overhead. Fasten it with an apparatus specifically designed for that purpose. It will be easier to use on the horse and eliminate the possibility of tripping or a hoof tearing the hose.

For a grooming stall, built-in recesses keep necessary tools nearby while keeping the environment safe. Consider a niche built for your horse vacuum or a built-in vacuum that connects to an internal unit, much like a house vacuum system. A collapsible saddle rack and hook in or near the wash stall and grooming stall can be handy.

Choosing the right flooring to meet your needs is often a matter of balancing what is wanted with what is affordable. Knowledgeable horse owners know that no stall flooring is perfect, so make sure you can live with any disadvantages. You want a surface that gives, is non-skid and durable, does not retain odor and is easy to clean. Mats in the stall offer the easiest cleanup option and can cut down on bedding requirements, but they can only be used on flat surfaces such as wood, concrete, asphalt or leveled stone dust.

Inside the barn, you want good lighting for ease of work and general good cheer. If the climate allows, skylights, transparent panels or openings on the upper sides of the walls can provide natural light. Not only does good light make cleaning easier, if the vet comes to care for a stall-bound horse, having a well-lit environment is an advantage.

When selecting hardware, whether for inside the barn or on gates or fencing, single-hand operation is considered to be the best. Latches that can be opened or fastened with one hand while leading a horse or carrying a bucket with the other are an important feature. They should also be durable enough to withstand the elements, years of use and horses leaning on them. Thinking ahead to everything you need in your barn and identifying a place for it will mean less clutter. You will also save time if you don't have to hunt for needed items. With function, efficiency and safety in mind, you can build a new barn or renovate an existing one to provide a better environment for your horse and also enable you to save time and effort in the future.

Barn Safety

In their natural environment, horses sometimes meet with challenges that lead to physical injuries, illnesses and sometimes death. For the modern, domesticated horse, conditions are very different from those of living in the wild, but, they, too, are exposed to conditions that can lead to injury, illness, and death unless owners are proactive in ensuring their safety.

Although horse owners would like to think that their horses are better protected from injury and illness than a horse in the wild, this very mind set can lead to catastrophic losses because of the very nature of the way horses are confined in barns and stalls and exposed to humans and other horses and animals.

Quite often, little thought is given to up-keep and safety checks of barns. Since barns pose safety hazards to horses, owners, workers, and visitors, a little time and effort can lessen or eliminate hazards and create a safe place for both animals and people. Maintaining a safe, healthy barn is of paramount importance to a horse owner, not only for the protection of horses and owners, but for the protection of everyone coming onto the property where accidents and exposure to illness and toxic substances can and do happen.

Prevention of injury

While no one likes to think of injuries and death, agricultural enter-prises, including equestrian-related facilities and farms, are among the most hazardous workplaces. Although accidents with machinery and vehicles account for over half of fatalities, falls, fire, structural inadequa-cies, horse-related injuries, and respiratory diseases are legitimate concerns for the horse owner.

Common sense should be used whenever working with machinery and vehicles. All machinery and vehicles should have regular safety checks. Horse trailers should be kept clean and in good repair, and safety proce-dures should be in place for both loading and unloading horses. Tractors, three-wheelers, and other small transport vehicles should be ridden and used only by those with the respect and know-how to safely operate the

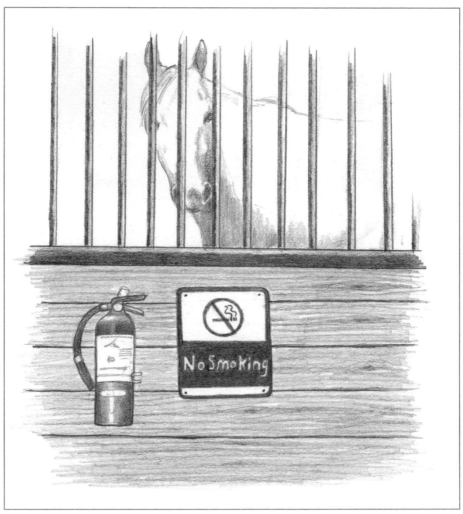

The safety consideration

Reducing the chances of injury to your horse, yourself and your barn visitors should be a primary concern of your healthy barn.

equipment.

Many barn injuries are the result of slipping or falling, with the most common site for a fall being the hay loft. Unstable pieces of equipment allowed to remain in the horse area, or slippery or uneven floors are a close second. Anything, from a dropped horseshoe to a piece of fencing wire carelessly thrown against a wall, can cause more damage to horse or human than can be imagined.

All floors should be kept clean, dry, and in good repair to prevent slips or falls. Ropes, pitchforks, tack, and other equipment should be kept off floors and in their proper storage areas when not in use. If the barn has plank floors, any loose, uneven, or worn boards should be either replaced or repaired.

All clutter, debris, and trash, both inside and outside of the barn should be cleared away at all times. Keep your barn clean of dust, cobwebs, oily rags, etc. which are unsightly and also are fire hazards.

Keep grooming and wash stalls clean, well-drained, and located in an open area to prevent wet, slippery floors. Keep watering troughs and lines in good repair and ensure floors are kept dry. Wearing slip-proof footwear, helmets (when needed), and functional clothing that stays close to the body will help prevent many injuries.

One absolute rule that everyone should follow is to put all equipment back where it belongs promptly after each use. Both humans and horses may get caught or hurt themselves on equipment, objects, or tack that is carelessly left in inappropriate places.

Fire safety

Fire is the greatest catastrophic threat to a barn. A few simple precautions can protect your barn and horses. Install a lightening rod, enough electrical outlets to avoid overloading, and modernize your circuit breakers. Don't store hay, bedding and other combustibles in the barn. Use recesses to accommodate items such as fire extinguishers. Protect electrical wires with rodent-proof conduit metal or hard plastic. Smoke from a fire causes eye irritation and respiratory damage. Depending on the concentration of smoke, successful evacuation from a burning barn can be extremely difficult given the frightened state of animals and the possible disorientation caused by inhaling smoke and carbon monoxide. Keep a halter and lead rope on every stall door. In a fire or other emergency, being able to lead your horse to safety is of maximum importance.

Smoking should be banned within 50 feet of barns and stables. Fire extinguishers should be located at every exterior door and next to the main electrical panel box. Install industrial-type heat and carbon monoxide detectors with a loud external siren or alarm. If you must use extension cords, use those with the best safety rating available and check them regularly to make sure wires and plugs are in good condition with no frayed or exposed wires.

Provide at least a 50 foot firebreak around your barn and post phone numbers of your veterinarian, fire department, and other emergency services in an accessible and visible place. Ask your fire department to do a walk-through of your barn and point out any corrective measures that should be taken.

Barn and stable layout should be safety-oriented, with exits clearly marked in case of emergency. Ceilings should be 8 to 12 feet high and door frames a minimum of 8 feet high and 4 feet wide for easy ingress and egress. More than one exit should be provided in all cases. This is especially important in the event of a fire when horses and humans may panic and become disoriented.

Accident prevention

Horses should be respected as the large animals they are. No shouting or running should be allowed in the stable or barn areas. Never assume a horse heard or saw you approaching and don't touch a horse unexpectedly. A swift kick may be the result.

Never allow children to play unattended around barns or stables and make sure a responsible adult is present to monitor children in these tempting, but dangerous, areas. In addition, keep all equipment and machinery properly stored and out of the way to prevent tripping or other accidents to horses and humans.

> ## Danger
> ### Avoiding the most deadly accidents
>
> Accidents with machinery and vehicles, especially tractors, account for over half of farm and ranch fatalities. Most tractor accidents resulting in fatalities are due to roll-over. Don't allow anyone to drive a tractor or operate equimpment without proper training, and always use safety belts to avoid roll-over injuries.

Since clutter contributes to accidents to both horses and people, it should be kept to a minimum at all times and any horse care items or tools should be put back in the proper place daily.

Barn tools and equipment

Although horses in their natural setting historically, have been able to exist and sometimes thrive without the modern conveniences that horse owners now have, caring for the domesticated horse by its very nature is much easier, healthier and more cost effective with the proper tools and equipment. Depending on your situation, you may choose to go with minimal equipment when caring for your horses. The necessary tools and equipment for a healthy barn break down into several categories including: mucking and cleaning supplies such as shovels, rakes, muck rakes, muck buckets, brooms, and brushes; a wheel barrow, feeding and watering equipment including buckets, locking feed bins, water buckets or tanks; stall mats, blanket bars or hooks near stalls.

Cleaning and mucking tools

First on the list of tools you need in your barn and stable area are those for cleaning and mucking out stalls. Horse stalls need to be mucked out every day to prevent waste from building up and disease from spreading. Tools for cleaning include a shovel which can be used for many things. In addition to the shovel you will want a wide tooth pitch fork which will come in handy when working with bedding as well as with hay. With a wide tooth pitch fork you can lift a heavy pile of bedding easily. Also look into scrubbing brushes, hoses and buckets for periodically washing out the stable and barn.

A special manure scoop comes in handy in every horse barn. The special scoop allows you to scoop up horse waste without removing all the bedding that is still clean. The small tines of the manure scoop will slide right through the bedding to pick up the manure. A garden rake can be used to clean out the barn walkways and stalls. You can rake fine materials up with ease and use it to help move around bedding and hay when necessary. You will also find many other uses for this tool. When it comes to cleaning water buckets or tanks and feed bins, a regular toilet brush works well especially in cold weather when you may not want to get your hands wet.

In addition, one of the best labor saving devices you can own is a muck-bucket cart. Because wheelbarrows can be so awkward and are hard to dump, a muck bucket is a good solution. It can be moved with only one hand, which leaves your other hand free to carry the other necessary tools.

Feeding and watering systems

Next to keeping the barn and stable clean, having the necessary items for feeding your horse is important. In addition to the pitchfork for

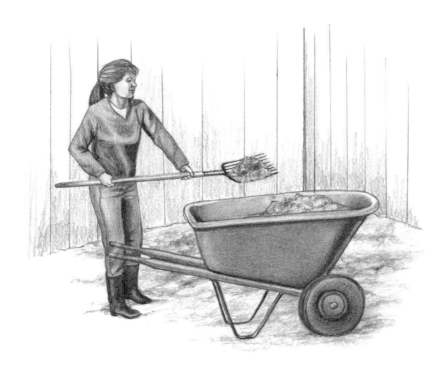

Keeping ahead of the mess

We have all visited dirty and smelly barns. The best way to avoid your barn becoming the same is to develop a daily, weekly and monthly schedule for cleaning and maintenance.

getting flakes of hay to your horse, having a grain bin or container that has a locking lid so that your horses are not able to open it is important. A grain bin will also keep the grain safe from other animals such as cats, dogs and raccoons. Along with a grain bin, you need a grain feeding utensil or feeding bag. Any feed store will have a variety of options for feeding grain.

To feed your horse hay, you will need a dry spot where the horse will not walk. If your horses keeps a tidy barn, you can feed them on the ground, but some horses are very messy and will poop anywhere. For these horses you will need an elevated hay manger or a hay bag. Although it is usually best to store hay out of the barn and stable area for fire safety, having easy access to the hay is important and in some cases you may have an exterior opening through which you can pitch the hay to make it convenient to carry to horse stalls.

Feed tubs or buckets that are detachable are very useful. Because of the differences in the behaviors of horses, you need to be prepared for those that are messy eaters as well as those that are neat eaters. If all of your feed tubs are detachable, you can clean them whenever needed.

Since horses need a steady supply of clean fresh water for good health, having buckets, waterers, or water tanks that are easy to clean and care for is important. If your horses spend most of their time in pastures or paddocks, water tanks in those areas may suffice along with water buckets for use in stalls. If your horse spends much of its time in the stall, having a stall water supply is essential. Some horses prefer to drink from buckets instead of automatic waterers. In either case, you will need to keep track of how much each horse is drinking to ensure good health.. Some horse owners that don't have water piped into stalls, find that using a hose reel saves time and effort. Buckets will need to be filled every day at a minimum, and it becomes quite tedious to drag a hose down an aisle and back again or carry buckets to a central spigot. A hose reel allows you to bring the water where it is needed effortlessly and makes the process much easier. Some horse owners use bucket hooks on their buckets to limit the strain when lifting heavy buckets. These are C-shaped, and they don't need to be snapped closed. The handle simply fits into them and is held secure.

For horses in cold climates, a water heater for horse drinking water is important. It will keep water from freezing over and at a temperature comfortable for the horse to drink which means better health for the horse. The heaters can be used in stock tanks where the horses are outside or you can shop for smaller heaters for in stall use. Make sure that the electrical outlets are protected and that horses cannot get to them.

Keeping barn and stable air healthy

Experts agree that a proper ventilation system is an important consideration in horse barns and stables, but many times it is overlooked. Not only do horses have dusty bedding, they urinate and defecate on the floor, and have a need for a stream of fresh air into their stables for health reasons.

Since natural breezes can move most of the air in a stable, every barn needs a minimum of two sets of openings throughout the horse-occupied area to allow air to enter and exit. During cold weather, the warmer, stale air inside rises and escapes through the upper openings.

Fans properly placed on the ridge line of the building or in other places can pull out stale, moist air and pull in fresh air through the overhang or the windows. Multiple openings are needed for efficiency.

Handling and feeding animals can create air quality problems with dust and other contaminants in your barn. Installing floors that are as self-cleaning as possible can help reduce dust. Keep ventilation systems in top working order by cleaning all vents and providing good circulation of air. Barn fans and vents require routine maintenance and cleaning for maximum efficiency.

Handy general-care tools and equipment

A well planned barn and stable area will also have areas for cross tying of horses, wash racks, and tack storage. Blanket bars in convenient places near stalls or on stall doors means you can keep blankets, fly masks and boots, as well as other every day needs readily accessible, allowing you to reach up and grab something without having to walk to the other side of the barn. Many horse owners find stall mats to be an important item. Use of rubber mats mean that the horse requires less bedding, and they are also easy to clean. In addition, the mats give horses a comfortable, smooth surface on which to stand which can be an improvement over standing on the bare floor of the stall.

Having the necessary tools and equipment for your horse barn and stables in convenient, easily accessed areas will save time, effort, and allow you to spend more time enjoying your horse whether actively longeing it for exercise, watching it in turnout or riding for pleasure, all of which give the horse the activity and movement necessary to good health.

Housekeeping

In their natural environment, housekeeping for horses is negligible. By nature horses are fastidious animals, keeping their waste away from their food sources and keeping themselves clean by rolling in dirt or vegetation when they feel the need for it. Domesticated horses, especially those that spend most of their time in stalls are a different story. An average 1,000 pound horse produces around 54 pounds of manure daily, along with quantities of urine, and soiled bedding. This means that stalls should be mucked and cleaned daily to minimize pests and keep horses clean and dry along with maintaining air that is free of dust and odors, especially ammonia.

Odors in barns and stables can become intense, especially during cold months when doors and windows are closed to keep the cold out. Sunlight is a critical component for keeping odors at bay. Gases from urine thrive in dark, damp areas and the result is the pungent odor. Whenever possible, maximize the amount of sunshine let into your barn. Dutch doors are good too because they allow in low air and sunlight at the same time.

Floor coverings, such as mats and grids, reduce the amount of labor involved in stall cleaning in two ways: by facilitating drainage and by reducing the amount of bedding needed. Properly installed, graded mats or grids can channel urine to a drain or through the floor, eliminating the hours you've been spending each month digging out wet spots. They'll also protect floors, cutting down on or eliminating the heavy work of repairing holes or uneven surfaces each year. Mats have one additional advantage: Since they provide cushioning, they require less bedding on top.

A better approach to barn house keeping tasks

In addition to waste containment and removal, it is important to have a systematic approach to housekeeping in all horse-related areas similar to the approach for maintaining the homes where people live. Housekeeping tasks can be designated as daily, weekly, monthly, seasonally, biannually or yearly depending on the number of horses, horse-related activities, and the general nature of barns, stables, paddocks and pastures.

> ### Note
> #### Mountains of manure
>
> Storing and disposing of manure is an ongoing challenge. Keep the manure pile contained, and far enough away from the paddock and barn areas to reduce flies. Your local cement company may have available large concrete blocks made from excess concrete available. These block weigh a ton or more, but can be fitted together to build a partially enclosed manure pile.

Daily tasks should include checking and cleaning all water buckets, feed bags and utensils. This works best if it is a priority related to the regular feeding and water of the horse. Keeping feed storage areas and grain bins clean and rodent proof requires checking on a regular basis, usually at least once a week.

Establishing an organized cleaning system helps save time and effort. Clean stalls from front to back, back to front or side to side, It doesn't matter what your pattern is; just stick with one method for more effi-

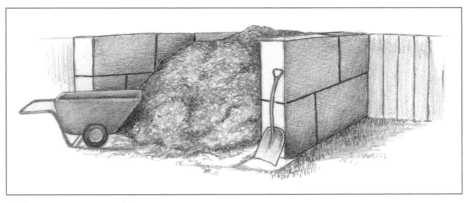

The manure pile

Horses produce prodigious amounts of waste. Creating an area for manure storage will reduce the fly population, and facilitate composting or later disposal.

ciency. Simplify waste removal by placing a tarp outside the stall door and tossing everything into the center. When the tarp is full, pick it up by the corners and place it in the wheelbarrow or carry it to the manure heap. Some horse owners prefer a manure cart over a wheelbarrow because it is easier to guide with one hand on the way to depositing the manure. Sloping floors can help with drainage and make cleaning easier.

In general, all physical areas of barns and stables should be hosed down or cleaned at least twice a year; more often, if they become dirty or cluttered. A good general cleaning in the spring and again in the fall before winter sets in works well in most areas.

Cleaning of tack should be done either after every use or on a weekly or monthly basis depending on how often it is used. Blankets, fly sheets, and pads should be cleaned and aired whenever needed, but at least several times a year for better wear and horse health.

Inspection and repairs to barn and stable structures, fences, and other horse-related areas and equipment are an important part of good house keeping and should be made as soon as any breakdown or weakening occurs. By being alert to changing conditions such as the deterioration of a fence post or a latch that fails to close on a stall door, a horse owner can stay ahead of the game. If not made promptly, small repairs can grown into major, costly and dangerous situations. A proactive horse owner can save money, time and effort by keeping barns, stalls, fences, tools and equipment in tip-top shape through good housekeeping.

Fencing

Fencing serves three main purposes: keeping horses where they belong, providing safety, and adding aesthetic value. How much importance is placed on each function depends on the owner's budget, the value of the animals, and priorities. Many horses are extremely valuable and that justifies the extra cost of building a fence that is safe, strong and attractive.

Horses are athletic and more apt to jump a fence if it is too low. According to experts, the minimum recommended height for perimeter pasture fences for horses is 5 feet. This height will deter most horses from attempting to jump and will also reduce the temptation for people to reach over the fence to pet or feed horses. A 5 foot minimum height fence is both horse-safe and people-safe.

For paddocks or small pastures and turn-out areas fewer than 2 acres in size, corrals and stallion pens, a general rule is that the top of the fence should be at eye level with the horse's head in a natural upright position. This is usually 4 to 6 inches above the horse's withers. This height will discourage fighting over the fence and help prevent horses from leaning over the fence, although the sure way to eliminate leaning and rubbing on any fence is with an offset electric fence wire.

Determining the best fence for your situation

The kinds of fences commonly used for horses include rail made from wood or PVC, various forms of galvanized and vinyl coated wire, electric and combinations of these. Whatever the fence is made of, it needs to be highly visible, resistant to damage by horses, durable, attractive and safe for contact by horses. By looking at the fences in your area and doing some research either on line or at fencing supply stores, you will be able to determine which kind of fencing will work best for your and your horses in your particular circumstances.

Electric fences

Electric fences are very effective in controlling horses once the horse has encountered the fence, but good visibility is extremely important and is not a characteristic of electric fences built with smooth steel wire. To increase visibility, one or more strands of vinyl coated wire or high-tensile vinyl tape should be included in the fence.

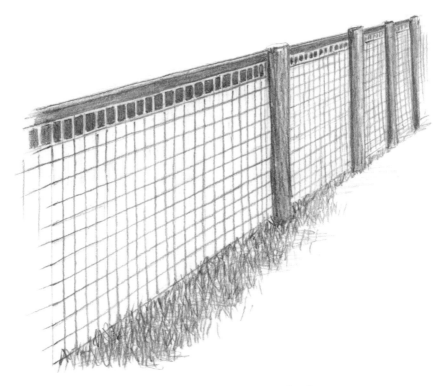

Good fencing a safety and liability priority

Fence related horse injuries can be crippling or fatal. Install or upgrade your fence to make it horse friendly and safe. Remember that you are liable for your horse and an escaped horse on a public road are often the causes of accidents and lawsuites.

One added advantage to electric fencing is that it does provide some protection from predators such as dogs, which sometimes like to chase horses. Once a dog has experienced an electric fence, he will not likely get close to it again. If a properly designed fence charger known as a "controller" or "energizer" is used, an electric fence is quite safe for use around animals as well as humans. While high voltages are used to shock the animals and cause them to avoid touching the wires again, the extremely short duration of the electric charge prevents damage to animals or humans.

An electric fence does require maintenance. Vegetation growing up around the wires reduces effectiveness. A large amount of contact will eliminate its effectiveness as the charge is shorted to the earth through the vegetation. It is important to be diligent to make sure that lightning or other power failures do not affected fence power.

A strand of electric fence wire can be added to a rail or wire mesh fence to increase the effectiveness and durability of the fence. If horses are damaging the fence by reaching over it to graze, a strand of electric fence across the top should prevent this. A strategically placed strand can also help by discouraging predators.

Waste management

When horses lived in their natural habitat in the wild, nature took care of waste management. Where horses were free to roam, horse waste did not accumulate into fly-attracting heaps. Nature took care of odors and made use of the nutrients left in the manure to keep the next generation of forage growing. Since horses are by nature fastidious , keeping waste away from forage and water sources was a natural way of taking care of business.

Under the best circumstances with only a few domesticated horses, the daily task of removing manure and stall waste takes time and energy. Add more horses or inclement weather conditions and this task becomes a problem, especially in areas with cold winters where weather conditions cause horse owners to accumulate a stack of horse waste.

Strategic planning for waste management

Proper management of manure and horse waste is a priority for maintaining a healthy barn. Internal parasites, insects, rodents, and odors can be manure related health concerns on horse farms. These issues can be minimized through carefully planned manure storage and handling. Internal parasites may be found in horse manure and can compromise the health and welfare of the horses stabled or grazing the land.

Composting manure and properly timed land application can limit the risk of parasite exposure. Insects, especially flies, become a nuisance on farms where stockpiled manure serves as the fly larvae habitat. Fewer flies will develop if you remove manure from the site or make it undesirable for fly breeding.

Rodents can be a problem when manure is stockpiled for extended periods of time, providing a warm, safe environment. Additionally, nuisance odor from manure piles can result in strained relationships with neighbors.

Many reasons exist for creating a temporary manure stack on a horse farm. It may be too wet to take manure to the field. It may be the only storage available on a small farm. Whatever the reason, consider the location carefully. Keeping the manure storage site screened with vegetation, fencing, or by location will help not only to enhance the beauty of your farm, but will lessen any chance for complaints about zoning violations by neighbors.

Conclusion

Whether you house your horse at your home or farm, or keep him at a commercial stable, the barn is the focal point of horse care. Your barn may be a simple as a lean-to shed, or as complex as an estate barn with living quarters. Regardless, the purpose and activities that make horse housing important and safe remain constant. Safety and promotion of good horse health are the concern of horse housing. In this chapter, you learned about common sense practices that can be implemented to keep your barn safe and healthy.

A properly designed barn considers maintenance and routine care activities. You have learned about the tools that make house-keeping easier, as well as how to select and place equipment such as waters and feeders that provide safety, and mimic the natural way of horse's feeding. Respiratory health requires excellent ventilation. Hoof health requires a relatively dry and sanitary stall floor. Runny eyes and noses, and some skin ailments result from too much dust. A truly healthy barn is a challenge.

Although most of us recognize the need for a barn structure, too few of us realize the importance of having our horses outdoors, in social groups, ideally grazing a natural forage. In a chapter devoted to healthy barn, the last point that we leave you with is to keep your horse outdoors, in the clean, fresh air as much as possible.

Top-5 takeaways

1. Confined horses are prone to injury. The number one concern for horse housing is providing a safe and healthy environment.
2. Horses generally prefer to live outside, but having shelter available for extremely cold, wet or dangerous weather is beneficial. Consider also the need for housing a sick or lame horse.
3. Horses are large animals and require sturdy buildings with oversized doors and high ceilings. Stall sizes should match the use of the stall and the breed of the horse.

4. Ventilation and sanitation are prime considerations. Fresh air reduces respiratory ailments and the cool air is appreciated by the horses. Clean stalls reduce the chance of disease or infection. In wet weather or during changes of season, hoof abscesses or allergies may result from unclean stalls.

5. A safe barn is a clean barn. Maintain paddocks free of debris and never store machinery around horses. Aisle should be kept clear and cleaning tools should never be left around horses or in barn aisles.

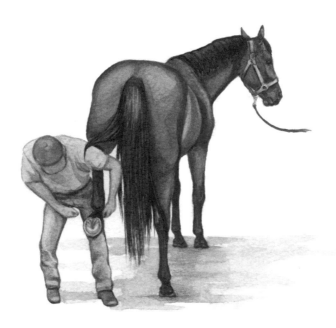

Chapter 7 Hoof Care

Introduction

Your well cared-for horse will rarely need a visit from your equine veterinarian. Your farrier, on the other hand, will be a fairly consistent visitor to your barn. Unfortunately, it is getting more and more difficult to find a farrier, Demographic trends and the physical demands of the trade have reduced the number of new farriers and the older experienced farriers are often not accepting new clients as they move toward retirement. Finding and keeping a skilled farrier is an important priority for the horse owner.

Virtually all domesticated horses require hoof care. Some require frequent hoof care; others require less frequent hoof care. How often your horse needs foot attention depends on the horse itself, along with what you ask your horse to do, the terrain in your barnyard and riding areas and more. Some horses can go months without farrier hoof care. Others require attention every 6-8 weeks, or even more often in some cases.

This chapter will help you understand the requirements for hoof care, what you can do and when you need the farrier. You will also learn how to find a good farrier and judge his or her performance. You will learn about common hoof diseases and conditions, what you can do and when you will need additional care from your farrier or your veterinarian.,

Do horses really need shoes?

In their natural state, when horses spent much of their time grazing and traveling over rough terrain, their hoofs usually wore down in a consistent manner in relationship to the way they moved and their level of activity. Hoof conditions are much different in domesticated horses that spend much of their time on artificial or man made surfaces in barns, stalls, arena and paths. Since the hoof is a vital part of the horse, and a healthy hoof is essential to the health, well-being, and usefulness of the horse, hoof care is a priority for most horse owners.

Genetics and hoof health

Genetics affect your horse's feet. If you purchase a horse from parents with mealy, soft feet, the odds are excellent that you will get a horse with a similar problem. Some breeds are well known for superior hoof health just as certain breeds and lines are noted for athleticism or temperament. In general, Arabians have tough, good feet. Morgans tend to have hoof problems, such as laminitis. In reality, you may not know much about your horse's family tree when it comes to feet, so you have to work with the hoofs you have.

The benefits of regular hoof care

Normally, the hoof wall grows at the rate of about three-eighths inch per month. Regular trimming is necessary to prevent sand cracks, quarter cracks, and breaking off of the hoof wall which can result in lameness. In addition, trimming maintains the correct length and hoof angle and balances the hoofs so a horse moves easily. A horse that receives regular hoof care is potentially a safer horse to ride, both for the rider and horse itself. The horse is less apt to slip, stumble, or fall. In addition, he is less likely to sustain injuries that would either put him out of service or require the services of a veterinarian.

Proper care of your horse's hoofs is basic economy. Allowing the feet to accumulate an excessive growth of wall may prevent the frog and elastic structures of the hoof from contacting the ground, thereby preventing the hoofs from performing their proper functions. It is important to keep in mind that horses' hoofs should be trimmed in such a manner as to keep them in a condition as close as possible to that which nature intended for the health of the horse.

Hoof care should begin on normal foals at approximately one month of age. As long as foot growth progresses normally, the foal should be trimmed approximately every four weeks. The feet should be kept level and the edges of the wall rounded to prevent breaking. In the normal foal this will correct bone growth in the hoof and limb. It is also important to keep flares from growing on one side of the hoof. This creates excessive stress on the bones and joints that may lead to lameness and incorrect bone growth.

Because of the basic nature of horses' hoofs, the concussive force they endure, and the susceptibility to injury and disease, basic hoof care is not only a necessity, but it can also save the horse owner time and money, and, in many times will quite literally save the life of the horse by preventing conditions that lead to lameness and death.

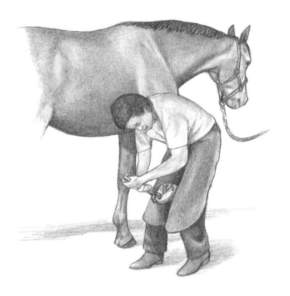

An important relationship
A good farrier develops a relationship with his client horses and owners. Pre-scheduled periodic visits for hoof healthcare are an important part of horse healthcare.

Hoof care as preventive medicine

Diseases such as thrush, navicular disease, and puncture wounds have devastating consequences if not caught in early stages and treated. A daily once-over including picking your horse's hoofs and making sure that they are in good condition will not only save your horse from pain and suffering, but will save you time, effort, and vet and farrier bills.

Weather and rain and other pasture conditions can lead to softening or cracking of horse hoofs, which can cause serious problems. When hoofs weaken from being too damp or too dry, cracks may occur, allowing infection-causing microbes to move deeper into the horse's foot.

A daily check-up of the hoofs can catch problems in their earliest stages thereby saving not only the horse's health, but farrier fees, also.

Caution
Be prepared for a foot emergency

Post the phone numbers of your veterinarian and farrier in your barn. When you leave your horses in the care of others, or if you should come across a serious injury, having these numbers near by can save you or a caretaker time in getting advice from your veterinarian or farrier.

However, knowing and having access to a competent farrier on a regular basis should be a priority for every horse owner. A farrier who is familiar with your horse will be able to nip problems in the bud in addition to making sure your horse has the hoof care necessary. Prompt treatment of hoof issues is vital to your horse's health.

Without a doubt, a horse's hoofs are one of the most important parts of the animal. Given a split hoof, nail prick, or stinky hoof, the first call should be to the farrier.

Farrier - specialized training and tools

Effective training to become a farrier is not easy or soft in any way. Actual experience working with horses under all kinds of conditions is necessary whether it is in the hot weather of August or the cold snowy conditions of February. In addition, a farrier must have a thorough knowledge of hoof diseases and structural problems and how they affect not only the hoof, but also the entire horse. Acquiring the skills a farrier needs to be successful in diagnosing all kinds of limb and hoof problems, trimming and balancing hoofs, choosing the best kinds of horse shoes for the particular horse and devising corrective measures where necessary is a time-consuming and difficult process.

In addition to the training a farrier has undergone, a professional farrier will have a tool kit of specialized tools and equipment to use in taking care of the horse's hoofs. These tools make the job easier, save time, and help keep the horse's hoofs properly balanced, healthy and in good condition.

Basic farrier tools

Hoof tester - A devise used in the examination of the horse's hoofs to pinpoint sources of pain by applying pressure in certain areas.

Farrier's rasp - This is a multi-purpose tool that all farriers use. It is like a nail file for horses and enables the farrier to keep the horse's hoofs even and level if unshod or lightly rasp any hoof that overhangs a shoe. It is used to finish a trim by rasping off any extra hoof and rounding up the edges. It can also be used to rasp down nails and hoof wall where needed.

Farrier's knife - The farrier uses this specialized knife to cut out excess sole and frog in the feet of the horse.

Hoof nippers - These are used to cut the hoof wall down to the correct length and to cut off any excessive or damaged sole or hoof area to reduce the need for extra rasping.

Horseshoe pullers - This tool looks like a hoof nipper, but is larger. It is used to pull off the horse's shoe or shoes when necessary.

Anvil - All farriers need an anvil to mold horse shoes into the proper shape and style needed. Since each horse's hoof is different, the farrier needs to custom fit each shoe by shaping it on the anvil.

Nailing hammer - A farrier's nailing hammer is a small hammer that is used to punch nails through the horse's hoof to hold the shoe in place. The one side is used to drive the nails and the other side, which has two protruding claws, allows the farrier to "wring off" the nail when it comes out the side of the horse's hoof.

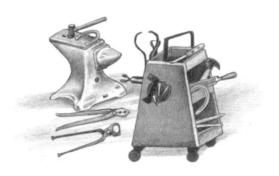

A farrier's trade tools

Simple but highly refined tools that have emerged from centuries of hoof care include: anvil, hammers, nail pullers, trimmers, hoof testers, files, rasps and more.

Nail clinchers - These clinchers are used to fold over the nail to make sure the horse shoe stays on the hoof. Two different kinds of clinchers are used. One has a short, ball-like head and the other an "alligator-like" head. Most farriers develop a personal preference for the one that works best for them.

Nailing or clinching block - This is usually a small piece of metal with an angled edge. It is put underneath the wrung-off nail when "setting" the nails before clinching.

Hoof stand - A hoof stand is used for finishing a nailing job and is especially helpful in easing the strain of lifting an injured leg. Hoof stands come in many heights and shapes and each farrier determines which kind works best in their practice.

Hoof gauge - Some farriers use a specialized gauge to measure hoof angles and check the balance of the hoof. This is a relatively new item in the farrier's tool kit and some farrier's prefer to used their eyes and their experience when determining hoof angles and balance.

> ## Note
> ### What tools do you need?
>
> You should invest in and learn to use a few simple tools that can be used in an emergency. 1) Hoof pick for obvious reasons; 2) A farriers rasp can be used to remove cracked hoof material. 3) A horse shoe puller to remove dangerously loose shoes.

For the most part, a farrier's skill, and knowledge plus the specialized tools and equipment used in hoof care are the horse owner's best insurance when it comes to keeping a horse's hoofs and lower limbs healthy and properly shod. After all, your horse's soundness largely depends on the health, stability, and balance of its lower limbs and hoofs.

Hoof care by the owner

Under natural conditions in the wild, research shows that wild and feral horses maintained "good" feet while living on rough, rocky ground. The biomechanics of the foot dictate that with movement, blood is pumped into the horse's feet increasing circulation and enhancing growth. This process occurred naturally as horses grazed through the day and into the night in their natural setting.

In wild and unshod horses, these activities allowed usage to wear away the hoofs and create calluses on the sole, with the layer of callus serving as a protective barrier against wounds and infection.

Because of the importance of healthy, well-maintained hoofs in domestic horses that live under very different conditions, a responsible horse owner pays attention to the state of the horse's hoofs on a daily basis. By careful assessment of hoof conditions, you will be able to save time effort and money on farrier or veterinary bills.

Most horse owners know the importance of picking and cleaning the horse's hoofs before and after each ride, or at least a couple of times a week.

What to look for

While picking out any small rocks or objects, pay attention to what is going on with each hoof. Is the temperature and pulse normal? Does the frog have a firm texture, without any indication of problems? Note any signs of injury, including punctures. Sniff the horse's feet to make sure that no bad odors are present, indicating thrush or other infections.

Checking your horse's pulse at the palmar digital artery which is located at the posterior (back) groove behind the suspensory ligament, just in front of the sesamoid bones in the middle of the fetlock is helpful in assessing foot health.

This pulse is more intense when there is increased blood flow to the foot, normally from exercise or abnormally from pain or inflammation. This artery is not commonly used to determine the pulse rate but it is very important in assessing foot problems, such as abscesses, laminitis, or other causes of foot inflammation.

The normal pulse rate ranges from 32 to 52 beats per minute, but it is the intensity that is most helpful in determining pain or inflammation. An easily felt equine digital pulse is commonly called a bounding digital pulse. The sensation is like a throbbing headache or an injured finger. It is not an increase in speed, but instead an increase in strength.

If your horse is shod, check the shoes on a regular basis, even if the horse is more of a pasture ornament and isn't ridden often. Make sure all nails are in the correct position and that the shoe isn't loose, pulling away, or shifting position. Call the farrier whenever you see problems with the shoes.

Additional considerations

Make sure your horse's diet provides the best possible hoof health. Check with your veterinarian or farrier to see if the diet is adequate or if a change in feed or the addition of supplements would be helpful.

If you are hauling the horse to shows, events, or for trail rides, protect the horse's hoofs by using proper bandages or boots. Several good options are available, including bandages and boots with Velcro fasteners for easy application and removal.

Don't allow your horse to spend time standing in mud, wet grass, boggy pasture, or unsanitary, urine-soaked bedding. These conditions lead to swelling and softening of the hoofs, which may allow the nails of the horseshoes to loosen.

When wet conditions are followed by dry conditions, the hoofs will split or crack, leading to discomfort and providing a pathway for infections that may lead to abscesses. In addition, a horse that is left standing in mud or boggy pasture may develop thrush or scratches that can lead to lameness.

Work with your farrier by scheduling regular visits. Once a farrier gets to know the horse's needs, a timetable of visits can be worked out to make sure hoof health is an ongoing priority.

In many cases, a capable farrier will be willing to instruct the horse's owner in day-to-day care of the hoofs and shoes to maximize care without straining the budget or time schedules of those involved.

Since horse's hoofs take a beating on a daily basis, every horse owner should be prepared for emergencies when a veterinarian or a farrier is not immediately available to deal with hoof issues that might affect the future soundness of the horse.

Some horse owners find that having hoof testers to help pinpoint points of infection or pain in the horse's hoof not only come in handy, but can help determine whether or not a call to the farrier or veterinarian needs to be made. Your regular farrier can explain the uses of hoof testers and show you how and where to use them.

Your farrier may be willing to train you in taking basic care of your horse's hoofs in an emergency, but be aware that the work is challenging and can be dangerous when it comes to working with large, sometimes cantankerous animals that may bite and kick when they don't want anyone touching their hoofs.

As a horse owner, should you trim or shoe your own horse? Probably not. Professional farriers have undergone rigorous school training to learn hoof structure and proper techniques for care. Most have apprenticed with an experienced mentor. All have handled multiple horses with a large variety of problems. You are far ahead to use an experienced professional in keeping your horse's feet in good condition.

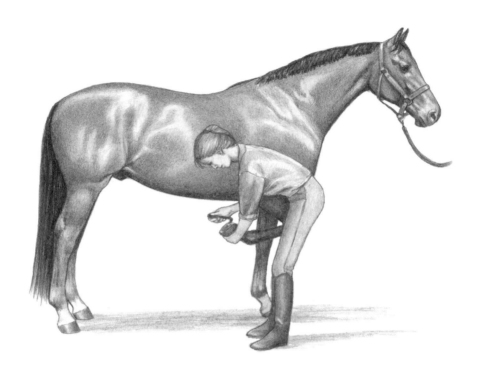

An owner's responsibility

Farriers can take care of periodic trimming and shoeing (as required), but it is up to you to check and clean your horse's prior to riding, and periodically (at least weekly) for horses that are not ridden.

Hoof care by the farrier

Routine hoof care is a part of every equine's life. In a natural environment, a horse's hoofs are maintained by the daily activities of the animal.

Domestic horses often need horseshoes because their hoofs harden less than in the wild and their circumstances do not provide adequate natural wear to maintain healthy hoofs.

A knowledgeable and well-trained farrier is a specialist in equine hoof care and has a working knowledge, not only of the anatomy and functions of the horse's hoofs, but also needed veterinarian skills to use in adequately caring for the horse's feet. The skills of a blacksmith are also necessary in making, applying and adjusting horseshoes.

An experienced farrier will have sound background knowledge of the practice of the craft along with experience in shoeing all types of hoofs, making shoes to fit all types of horses and working conditions, and also will be skilled in developing treatments to compensate for faulty limb action or form.

The many roles of the farrier

Farriers maintain the horse's hoofs by keeping them trimmed using tools such as rasps and nippers to cut away hoof material. Trimming helps maintain foot balance by keeping the feet at the proper shape and length. They also clean the feet and cut out excess hoof walls, dead sole and dead frog.

Farriers apply horseshoes as a corrective measure to improve the horse's gait and to help it gain traction when walking in slippery conditions such as ice. Farriers also design and apply shoes for race and performance horses according to the specialized needs of the individual horse.

Acting as a blacksmith, the farrier removes old shoes, trims the hoofs, measures shoes to the feet and bends the shoes to the proper shape before applying them.

Acting as veterinarians, farriers care for hoofs by watching for signs of disease or other ill health. They also watch for potential lameness issues, intervening before problems occur.

Horse owner and farrier as a team

Farriers appreciate the cooperation of the horse's owner and are likely to do their best when they have a sheltered, safe location with suitable cross ties for holding the horse while they do the necessary work. In addition, the horse should be ready and waiting when the farrier arrives. Horse owners who have trained their horses to stand and give their feet are very much appreciated.

Farriers usually welcome questions and are happy to explain why they are doing a particular procedure to the horse owner, although a good farrier is busy and may not have much time for chit-chat.

Like veterinarians and doctors, most farriers expect payment at time of service unless previous arrangements have been made.

Given the training and experience of a capable farrier, any problems related to the hoofs of the horse will be met head-on, increasing the productivity and enjoyment of both horse and owner. While the owner or handler may be involved in day-to-day care of the horse's hoofs and may learn how to do some trimming, a competent farrier should be part of the equation.

As a service based industry, farriers must combine technical competence with horsemanship and the ability to deal with clients. They appreciate horse owners who value their time and competence and establish a schedule of regular visits based on the horse's situation to keep hoofs healthy and prevent serious hoof problems before they develop.

> **Note**
> *Beware of "specialized" hoof trims*
>
> Natural or barefoot methods of trimming a horse's hooves are popular with many horse owners. These methods attempt to shape the horse's hoof in a manner consistent with the natural wear patterns observed in wild horses. Unfortunately, the footing conditions for your horse are probably different from those of a wild horse, so these particular trim styles may not be best suited to your horse or terrain. Let your farrier decide the best style of trim based on your horse's use and the local terrain.

"The farrier's craft takes years to master -- even a lifetime. And, about the time you think you understand it, your body is worn out!" Dr. Doug Butler

How to judge your horse's foot condition

The over-all health of a horse often rides on healthy hoofs. The horse's ability to run, jump, work, participate in competitions, trail rides, and interact with you and other horses all depend on the health of its hoofs.

Weather, environment, riding terrain, turnout frequency, horseshoes, heredity, and nutrition all affect equine hoof health

A horse owner needs to be aware of what a healthy horse's hoof looks, feels, and smells like to appraise the horse's hoofs on a regular basis. In addition, knowing each particular horse's hoofs is important in catching any unhealthy conditions before they become major problems.

While picking out any small rocks or objects, pay attention to what is going on with each hoof. Is the temperature and pulse normal? Does the frog have a firm texture, without any indication of problems? Note any signs of injury, including punctures. Sniff the horse's feet to make sure that no bad odors are present, indicating thrush or other infections.

Every horse owner or rider should know what healthy horn wall, sole, and frog, look like to be able to make informed choices over hoof care.

Environmental factors affect hoof growth

According to Steve Kraus, head of the Farrier Service at Cornell University's Large Animal Clinic, "There are also environmental factors that will affect hoof growth. Horse hoofs tend to grow faster with increasing daylight." So while your horse's hoofs may seem to stop growing over the winter months, that growth rate will increase during spring and summer months.

Dry, wet? Rocky, soft? Cold, hot? Summer, winter? Environmental factors affect hoof growth and condition all year. The amount of moisture your horse's feet are exposed to can also influence growth. If conditions are too wet, hoofs will get soft and become prone to sole abscesses and fungal infections. If there is too little moisture, hoofs may get dry and brittle. Try to keep stalls clean and provide mud-free areas for your horse in turnout areas.

No such thing as a perfect hoof exists in the real horse world. Horses' feet differ vastly from horse to horse. There may be the perfect hoof for the individual horse, meaning the horn is healthy, the connection with the coffin bone is tight and strong, the balance of the hoof matches the rest of the horse's body and allows for maximum movement, and the size of the hoof is ample for the size of the horse, but that specific hoof might not be at all perfect for another horse.

In addition, a functional hoof may serve the horse, but may not necessarily be healthy throughout or be optimal for the horse. Horse's hoofs change all the time relative to the weather, the time of year, the diet or the amount of exercise.

What a healthy hoof looks like

When looking at your horse's hoofs the wall horn should be smooth and growth rings, hardly visible. It has a natural and shiny coating almost looking a bit like lacquer unless the horse is exposed to rough terrain. No chips or cracks are visible and all horn tubules run in a straight line parallel toward the ground.

The outside of the wall protects against the environment, while the softer inner wall can flex and give and accommodate the somewhat flexible connection with the coffin bone.

The inner wall horn is produced by the lamellae that also produce the white line horn. As the outer wall grows down from the top, the inner wall constantly grows from the lamellae outward and joins the outer wall horn.

In a healthy hoof, the thickness of the wall is adequate all the way around the hoof capsule. In strong wall horn, the outer wall or pigmented wall is quite thick in comparison to the inner and unpigmented wall.

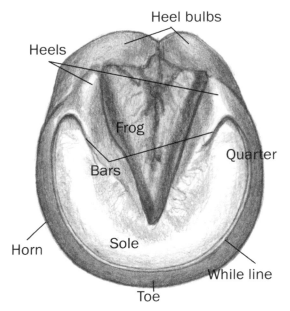

The white line of the hoof is really is not white at all, it is usually a cream or yellowish color. It is much less dense than wall horn as it is made up of the horny lamellae produced by the laminar corium. A healthy white

Structures of a healthy foot

As viewed from the bottom, your horse's foot should be symmetrical with well developed frog and bars. Purplish discolorations of the sole may indicate bruising, and a nasty smell may indicate thrush.

line is extremely narrow, not much over 1/16th of an inch, is uniform in color and is tightly connected to the sole and wall horn.

Usually, the white line can be judged only during trimming. As soon as the wall grows out, the white line horn can look much more distorted, and the color is often not visible.

The sole horn differs from the wall horn. Healthy sole horn of what is called the live sole plane appears smooth and uniform in color, except for hoofs that have a pigmentation pattern like striped hoofs. Sole keeps shedding constantly, and dead sole manifests as a cracked layer which covers the live sole plane.

Depending on terrain, amount of movement and frequency of trimming, there may be a lot of dead sole accumulated or none at all. Flaky sole horn may also be due to fungal disease.

Sole horn grows from the sole corium, from papillae similar to the wall horn. Sole horn is a much softer material than wall horn, its consistency can be compared to hard rubber. The horn tubules are sometimes visible like little pores on the sole surface.

Healthy frog horn is like hard rubber, very resilient but strong, and very difficult to pierce with a sharp object. Often it's necessary to trim a bit off to determine if the horn is truly healthy as the frog keeps shedding an often rough and frayed appearing layer.

Healthy frogs can have lots of different appearances depending on moisture content, amount of movement and the terrain the horse is living on. It can appear leathery and textured, or rubbery and totally smooth, may look very plump or a little shriveled, and it may have different colors.

> ## Note
> ### Preventing unhealthy hoof conditions
>
> The number one activity to guarantee hoof heath for your horse is to routinely inspect and clean the feet. The common hoof pick is inexpensive, and with a little practice -- easy to use. When you pick your horse's hoofs, look for thrush, cracks, asymmetrical wear and any other conditions mentioned in this section. Early detection and correction will save your horse potential pain and save you money by avoiding more costly treatments.

The shape of the hoof can give a good deal of information regarding the health of the foot, but many factors can affect hoof shape. Largely, the shape of the hoof is determined by the shape of the coffin bone in roughly the front two thirds of the foot and the health of the lateral cartilages and the frog in the back third.

Also, the height of the foot is determined by the height of the coffin bone. Although we do want and of course need ample horn protection of this bone, we do not want excess, as the hoof capsule is cone shaped, and any extra material past the sole must necessarily apply lever forces against its own structure, be it in the toe, quarters or heels.

Coffin bones take on as many shapes as there are hoofs. No two hoofs are totally alike, and additionally shape is dependent on age, breed, shoeing- and trimming practices, disease, amount of movement and the conformation of the horse's limbs and body, as this often causes one-sided pressure on the hoofs and manifests in steeper or more flaring walls.

Coffin bones are really very small in relation to the size of the skeleton, and they easily deform under pressure, never being able to return to their original shape. While a healthy coffin bone appears triangular when viewed from all angles, this shape can easily get distorted.

Also, front coffin bones usually have less concavity than hind coffin bones, but even that fact can get turned around at times by very poor balance, neglect or disease.

When viewed from the front, healthy hoofs appear quite short in height (the camera angle can cause lots of distortion again), the coronary band looks totally horizontal and straight, and the side walls are more or less angled toward the ground, but are quite straight without noticeable flares.

Truly healthy front feet have less concavity than the hind feet. Additionally, they also have a rounder shape than the hind feet, the frogs are usually not as wide and the distance between the frog and the toe wall is a bit longer.

Horse owners should realize that one style of trim is not correct for every horse. The only universal trim a horse could receive is one they would naturally produce living in the wild and constantly moving on different kinds of surfaces, as well as wading in streams and rivers.

In addition to the appearance of the hoofs, does the horse evidence pain when the hoofs are handled or hoof testers are used? How much exercise does the horse receive on a daily or weekly basis? Does the horse have a balanced diet based on its weight, nutritional needs and work load?

A horse that has foot pain, shorter stride than expected, starts out of the stall stumbling or stiff, but warms out of it when first ridden, potentially has a lameness problem or foot pain that needs to be investigated. Obviously, a lame horse needs to be evaluated by your veterinarian with consultation with your farrier.

When looking from the front or back of your horse, the ideal conformation is straight limbs that have feet evenly under the limbs for good support. Toed-in foot conformation is harder on a horse than toed-out foot conformation.

Feet that appear to have longish toes and low heels create more stress to the heels and the deep flexor tendon that wraps around the navicular bone and attaches to the bottom of the coffin bone.

One foot wider or narrower than the opposite front or hind foot potentially demonstrates that the horse doesn't bear equal weight on each side of its body. Obviously, any cracks or separations of the hoof makes normal trimming/shoeing more difficult no matter what the conformation. These can all be a direct cause for lameness.

Trained farriers and veterinarians are the best judges of horse hoof health and should be contacted whenever anything out of the ordinary appears to be happening with a horse's hoofs. A call to the farrier can often save time, effort, and money when it comes to nipping horse hoof problems in the bud.

Diseases and conditions of the hoof

Because horses are large animals with relatively fine limbs and hoofs, they are susceptible to many hoof diseases and conditions that affect their ability to live, work, and perform as horse owners expect.

In their natural state in the wild, horses did not have to bear weight, were not trained for intricate maneuvers involving limbs and hoofs, did not live on smooth, man-made surfaces, race on tracks, nor were they fed in ways that did not take into account the ways their digestive systems works best.

Instead, they moved from place to place through varying terrain that usually shaped their hoofs as nature intended while foraging for bits of food and fresh drinking water, often walking many miles per day.

Under present-day conditions, domesticated horses have an entirely different life. In addition, breeding for certain characteristics has made horses more susceptible to diseases and conditions that threaten the health of their hoofs and limbs.

Common conditions in horse's hoofs

It is important that horse owners check their horse's hoofs for sprung or shifted shoes, cracks, strange smells, or any other abnormalities after each ride or when it comes in from the pasture. Some conditions can be readily recognized by the horse owner, but others may need to be diagnosed by a veterinarian or farrier.

In addition to foot wounds and injuries that are common in horses, abscesses, hoof wall cracks, corns and bruised soles, and sheared heels are also common.

Puncture wounds are among the more serious wounds to a horse's foot. They can easily be contaminated and lead to serious infections causing lameness and other health issues. Lacerations to the coronet happen when a horse tangles with barbed wire, sheet metal or other objects.

An abscess is an infectious pocket within the hoof. Usually, this occurs after a foreign object, such as a nail or sharp stone, penetrates the hoof. If your horse has a hoof abscess, he will probably hold his leg up and be hesitant to put pressure on that foot due to the pain.

If the abscess is not drained, it can lead to bacterial laminitis, tetanus, septic arthritis or tenosynovitis, pedal osteitis, blood poisoning and destruction of the digital cushion or fracture of the navicular bone. Your veterinarian will open and drain the abscess; you will need to follow up with medication, poultices, soaking, or whatever else is prescribed.

> ## Note
> ### *Watch the feet*
>
> People experienced in high level horse competitions pay very close attention to the health and care of the horse's feet. Indeed, the angles, length of toe and heel, symmetry and overall condition of the feet shows the amount of care and attention devoted to this important topic.
>
> The more you learn about the care and importance of hoof health, the more you will pay attention to the foot care of horses that you see in your barn, on the trail and in the arena.

Hoof wall cracks occur when there is a separation or break in a hoof wall, Cracks are identified according to their location as toe, quarter or heel. Vertical cracks are classified as grass cracks or sand cracks. Large, deep cracks must be stabilized to prevent the hoof from splitting. Before stabilization takes place, the crack must be thoroughly cleaned and if moist or bleeding will require further care.

Corns and bruised soles are caused by rocks and other hard objects and usually involve the underlying sensitive laminae. A dry corn is characterized by red staining in the horn as a result of bruising or bleeding. Lameness is the most common sign of corns and bruises.

Sheared heels and quarters are often caused by improper trimming causing an imbalance. Sheared heels also predispose the horse to hoof wall injuries and thrush.

White line disease, also known as seedy toe, occurs when the white line disintegrates because of infection caused by bacteria, yeast or fungus. The infection begins at ground level and works its way up through the white line to the coronary band.

Thrush is a painful bacterial infection involving the frog. It is characterized by a putrid black discharge along with poor growth and degeneration of the horn.

Canker is a chronic infection of the horn tissues of the foot It begins in the frog and progresses slowly to involve the sole and sometimes the wall.

Contracted heels are a disorder where the foot of the horse is abnormally narrow or is actually contracted. This condition is caused by a lack of moisture in the foot, or by a lack a weight applied to the foot due to injury.

Quittor is a chronic, deep-seated infection of the lateral cartilages of the coffin bone. Injuries near the lateral cartilage are often the cause and a discharge via a sinus tract is often seen. During an acute attack the horse will be lame.

Sidebones occur when ossification of the lateral cartilages of the coffin bone occur allowing calcium to build up in the cartilage until it is converted to bone. Excessive concussion, improper shoeing, are primary factors in causing this condition.

Navicular disease is one of the most common causes of intermittent front leg lameness in horses. The foot stresses involved in activities with hard stops, twists at speed, abrupt changes in direction and forceful landings often affect both front feet.

Laminitis is a metabolic and vascular disease that involves the inner sensitive structures of the feet. Many causes of laminitis exist and one way the disease can begin is when bacterial endotoxins are released into the blood stream and directly affect blood flow into the hoof, causing inflammation of the sensitive lamina. Laminitis can also occur secondary to illness or gastrointestinal tract disease.

Acute laminitis is very serious and can begin suddenly with high fever and chills, sweating, diarrhea, fast pulse and rapid, heavy breathing. The digital artery at the fetlock has a pounding pulse and the feet are hot and painful. The horse alternately lifts one foot after another and gives evidence of severe pain when the foot of the sole is tapped.

Once signs of acute laminitis occur, it can be difficult or impossible to prevent permanent foot damage. Since acute laminitis is often brought on by the consumption of too much carbohydrates, consult your veterinarian without delay if you know or even suspect that your horse has ingested too much grain.

Treatment must be started before the signs of acute laminitis appear to be effective.

Chronic laminitis is diagnosed when laminitis persists for two days or more or when permanent damage to the foot occurs. A serious complication of laminitis is rotation of the coffin bone which is very difficult to treat.

Other complications of chronic laminitis include white line disease, thrush, separation of the hoof at the coronary band or sole and complete loss of the hoof. This is a brief summary of some of the diseases and conditions that affect horses. Responsible horse owners will always check their horse's hoofs and limbs on a regular basis and will call their veterinarian or farrier any time something out of the ordinary appears.

Use of hoof hardeners and bedding the horse on shavings or sawdust during wet weather or when the horse is being washed frequently, will harden the feet and prevent abscesses caused by foreign matter penetrating through the white line. When your horse's feet are properly trimmed and/or shod, the foot will land in a balanced way. This provides better circulation for the entire foot and encourages good hoof growth. A poor trim will hinder hoof growth. Functional strength instead of eye appeal should be emphasized for good hoof health.

Nutrition and hoof health

Good nutrition plays an important role in horse hoof health. If your horse is fed a balanced diet, complete with the necessary vitamins and minerals, its feet should be relatively healthy. For many horses, a diet that includes foraging for feed several times a day as in free choice feeding combined with regular exercise keeps circulation moving in the feet and helps maintain hoof health. Some horses may need supplements for maximum hoof health. Your veterinarian and farrier can help you determine if supplements are necessary for your horse.

Many nutritionists encourage the use of supplements for a horse that has poor hoof growth. Recommended supplements include zinc, calcium, protein (especially the amino acid methionine), and biotin. Zinc has to be added carefully and should be balanced with copper, calcium, and methionine to have any good effect. Calcium works in tandem with phosphorus, so you need the correct ratio there as well. You should consult

> ## Note
> *Biotin proven to increase hoof health*
>
> Researchers have found that hoof health and growth rate are improved when the supplement Biotin is added to the food. Biotin is a water soluble B vitamin that is actually produced in the horse's digestive tract. Research has shown that many horse's benefit from additional supplementation.

with your veterinarian and /or a nutritionist before you add any zinc or calcium to your horse's rations. Biotin and methionine are often supplemented in diets of horses that have slow hoof growth or hoof health issues.

The hoof is actually keratin, which is a protein similar to hair. So if your horse is protein-deprived, his hoofs will suffer. Keratin is also about four percent sulphur. Methionine, which contains sulphur and is a component of some proteins, is required to produce good-quality keratin. Lysine is another sulphur-based amino acid that helps with hoof growth. Both of these amino acids are found naturally in legume hays.

To learn more about horse health as it relates to nutrition, read the chapter on Nutrition.

Conclusion

This important chapter covered the basics of equine healthcare, with a focus on working with your farrier to establish excellent hoof and foot health. Feet and legs are injury prone, and can be subject to many conditions that are painful to the horse and take months for recovery. Preventative periodic hoof care will reduce the chances of injury or chronic conditions, and keep your horse in good form.

Fortunately, most non-working horses don't need shoes, and a trim is all that is required to keep the hoof growth and shape in check. Working with your farrier in developing a schedule for trimming or shoeing is the best way to get the best and most cost effective care that your horse needs.

In this chapter, you learned about the work of the farrier, and about your role in caring for your horse's feet. An attentive horse owner will learn to feel the legs and hoofs of the horse during daily or pre-ride care, and be able to recognize conditions that may lead to pain and lameness.

You also learned about various diseases and conditions that can occur in the hoofs, feet and legs of the horse. Recognizing the symptoms can help you keep ahead of a disease or condition, and prevent it from becoming more acute or chronic.

A great relationship with your farrier is important to the horse owner. It is becoming much more difficult to find and keep good farrier care, and you have learned in this chapter the importance of providing a proper work area for your farrier, as well as how to safely help your farrier when he or she visits.

The natural horse's survival depended on swift flight. Hoof and leg disease or injury leaves the natural horse exposed to predation. Fortunately, the roaming nature of the wild horse maintained their hoofs in trim and tough condition. Your challenge is to keep your domesticated horse's feet in proper trim and condition for his overall health and safety.

Top-5 takeaways

1. Your horse healthcare team generally consists of you, your veterinarian and a qualified farrier. All horses need periodic hoof care, and the farrier-horse relationship will save you money over the lifetime of your horse.

2. Healthy feet result from a clean environment along with frequent attention by the horse owner. You should "pick" your horse's feet prior to riding, or for those pasture ornament horses, at least weekly.

3. The period between professional attention depends on the use of the horse, the horse's hoof growth rate, and the overall health of the horse. For most horses, 6 to 8 weeks between trims is normal.

4. A host of diseases and conditions affect your horse's feet. Knowing how to identify and prevent these conditions is best for your horse and your pocketbook.

5. Good nutrition is important for healthy hoofs. For weak or slow growing hoofs, a biotin supplement may be helpful.

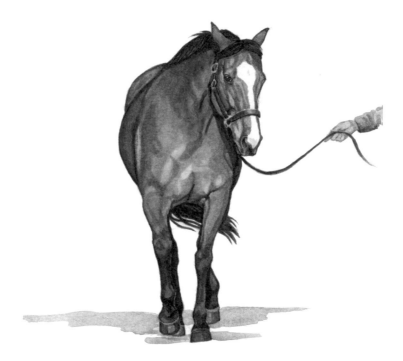

Chapter 8 Lameness

Introduction

Sooner or later, you will notice a slight limp or stiff motion in your horse - a signal that your horse is lame. Of all the diseases and conditions that horses suffer, lameness is the most common and potentially the most devastating. Because of this, we devote an entire chapter to this important topic. Simply defined, lameness is where the animal fails to travel in a regular and sound manner. Lameness ranges from very mild, where only an experienced observer that knows the animal can detect it, to very severe where the animal refuses to put any weight on the affected limb.

In this chapter, you will learn how to recognize lameness, and also grade the level of lameness as would your veterinarian. You will gain insight as to the causes of lameness, and also how you can avoid many causes of lameness through proper conditioning practices. In all but mild cases, your veterinarian should be called to provide a diagnosis and treatment. For mild lameness that does not resolve, your veterinarian should be consulted. Ignoring mild chronic lameness may result in painful arthritis that may be avoided with early diagnosis and treatment of the lameness.

Anatomy

The horse's anatomy has seen many changes down through the years since the first horse appeared. The longer legs with finely tuned structures of bones, ligaments, tendons and connective tissues developed through gradual changes and more recently have changed through breeding for certain characteristics in the horse's anatomy.

The hoofs have also gone through changes. The early ancestors of the modern horse walked on several spread-out toes, an accommodation to life spent walking on the soft, moist grounds of primeval forests. Eventually, the ancestors of the horse came to walk only on the end of the third toe and both side toes. A horses's leg conformation was critical to survival in the wild, and a horse's life depended on being capable of out-running predators.

In domesticated horses, good breeders focus on leg conformation to improve with each breeding. Proper leg angles place less stress on the joints, and the legs are better able to absorb the concussion from the impact of each hoof as it hits the ground. The front legs of the horse carry approximately 60 percent of the weight of the horse and are constantly subject to lameness with approximately 95 percent of lameness occurring from the knee down with the foot being the site of most problems. The hind limbs are involved in approximately 20 percent of cases of lameness, with the hock and stifle joints being the main problem areas.

A horse doesn't have a collar bone, so the front legs are not attached by joints, but rather to a sling of muscles and ligaments that support the weight of the horse and rider. The shoulder blade, or scapula, is connected to the spine by muscle and ligaments and allows freedom of movement and absorption of concussion. Since a horse's legs are made up of a finely tuned system of bones and joints, ligaments and tendons, muscles and connective tissue designed to carry a relatively heavy body, good conformation coupled with healthy limbs is extremely important for proper function. In addition, the legs of a horse must work together to support the horse as it stands and also to diminish compression during movement, thereby protecting the horse from injuries to its limbs.

Looking at the anatomy of a structurally sound horse, it is important to note that the horse has no muscles in its legs below the knees and hock. The lower part of the leg is made up of bone, tendon, ligaments, cartilage, skin and hair. For this reason, a great deal of consideration needs to be

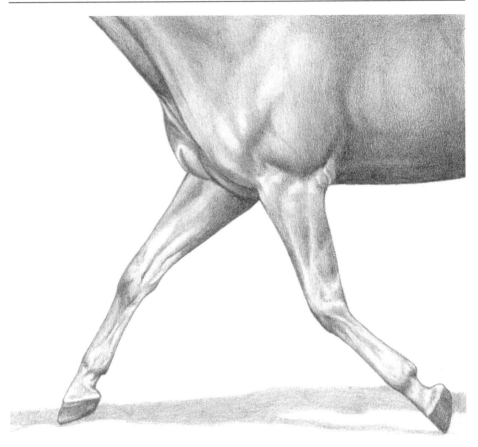

Nature's design

Your horse's legs are designed for running away from predators and covering large territories in search of food. Care must be taken to protect the fragile leg apparatus for horses that are ridden.

given to making sure that the legs of the horse are examined regularly so that any predisposition to unsoundness or injuries can be treated properly, thereby preventing lameness. Since the form of the horse's legs is closely associated with the function, it is not an overstatement to stress their importance as an extremely important part of the overall well-being of the horse.

Causes of lameness

Lameness is a common problem that affects nearly all horses. The most common causes of lameness are infections, traumatic injuries, degenerative and metabolic diseases, and developmental conditions. Determining the cause of lameness in a horse can be a daunting task for the best trained veterinarian. The history of the particular horse must be taken into account along with the circumstances surrounding the development of the lameness. What happened just before the lameness was noticed? Have the shoes been changed or has the hoof been trimmed recently? Was the horse ridden over uneven ground or possibly kicked by another horse?

Trauma as a cause of lameness

The limbs of a horse are subject to many kinds of injuries that vary from slight sprains to serious fractures. A sprain occurs when a sudden or severe twisting of a joint results in tearing or stretching of ligaments. A strain is usually less severe than a sprain and is the result of overstretching of ligaments or tendons through excessive use or improper movement. Sprains and strains are common injuries in the lower limbs of competition and performance horses and usually result from over loading or over stretching, but can also be due to a direct blow. The most common damages are to the tendons and ligaments that run from the knee down to the foot including the superficial digital flexor tendon, the deep digital flexor tendon and the accessory and suspensory ligaments.

Muscle strains caused by overuse or overstretching of muscle fibers in the croup and back of the thighs are another source of lameness. These usually occur during athletic competitions and the strain often includes ligaments and tendons.

Sore backs and loin injuries usually occur when horses are racing or jumping and somehow twist their bodies causing strain to the muscle groups. The involved muscles become firm, warm and painful, and the horse will have a shortened stride and gait alterations suggestive of hind-quarter lameness. Back injuries from falling or going over backward sometimes cause the spines in the back to impinge on each other or overlap. This often happens in the saddle area and may also affect horses without a history of back injury. The problem is most prevalent in hunters and jumpers, and horses with a swayed back are most commonly affected. Hind-quarter lameness and great sensitivity to pressure creating pain in the back are signs of overlapping or damaged spinous processes.

Fractures are another form of injury that are usually immediately recognizable, although in cases of some hairline and stress fractures especially those to the cannon bone and chip fractures involving the joints below the elbow and stifle or in the bones of the foot are not immediately obvious on visual inspection. Fractures are caused by accidents such as falls, being kicked by another horse, or stepping into a hole. Horses are also subject to compression fractures or fractures caused by high torque forces on a limb.

Bone fractures are usually classified as open or closed. An open fracture breaks through the skin and is readily observable. A closed fracture such as a simple fracture or a chip fracture is usually contained within the limb and becomes observable only when lameness, pain, swelling, or fever occurs. A hard fall or running into a solid object sometimes results in a fracture of shoulder or the spine. These types of fractures do not occur often because of the force necessary to fracture these larger, better protected bones. At one time, a diagnosis of a fracture meant either retirement or a death sentence for the horse. However, orthopedic techniques have advanced greatly and many fractures no longer carry a grim prognosis.

> ## Note
> ### Sticks and stones ...
> Horse's feet are tough and horses generally avoid stepping on sharp angular rocks when walking or trotting. When a horse canters or gallops, it is much more susceptilble to hoof injury due to stepping on sharp rocks. Help prevent a "stone bruise" by removing rocks from your riding areas, arenas, or trails where you canter, lope or gallop your horse.

Injuries to any part of the musculoskeletal system can result in lameness with tendon injuries being rather common in horses. Lacerated or ruptured tendons can occur in the legs and the feet usually from a deep cut, a fall, a kick from another horse, or damage caused by striking a stationary object. Tenosynovitis takes several forms depending on the location of the trauma and is distinguished by a sudden building of fluid within the sheath of the tendon accompanied by pain, heat and lameness.

Septic tenosynovitis is the result of bacterial infection resulting in pus and inflammatory enzymes that can digest the tendon. Pain and lameness are severe. Stringhalt involves the tendon of the lateral digital extensor muscle at the hock. It is characterized by a sudden upward jerking of the hind leg accompanied by an involuntary flexion of the hock as the horse steps forward. Some cases follow trauma involving the tendon, but in other cases, the cause is unknown.

Bursitis is the result of trauma to a bursa which is a closed sac lined by a membrane that secretes a lubricating fluid. These sacs are located between moving parts of the limb and act as cushions to prevent friction. An acute bursitis causes lameness. Bursitis affects shoulder joints, hips, the cunean tendon at the inside of the hock joint, the elbow, the knee and any other point of movement cushioned by a bursa, and is often evidenced by noticeable swelling in the area, as well as lameness.

Poor foot conformation, infrequent or inadequate hoof trimming resulting in a long toe and low heel, sheared heels, contracted heels and improper horse shoeing are thought to adversely affect the transfer of weight through the navicular complex to the ground leading to injury to the inner structures of the foot. Initially, lameness is mild with navicular disease and comes and goes. As lameness worsens, a stiff, shuffling gait with a shortened, choppy stride becomes characteristic making it difficult for the horse to function.

Rocks and other hard objects can bruise the sole or lead to corns that will cause the horse to limp with lameness getting progressively worse if not treated promptly. In addition, if a sole bruise resulting in an abscess is allowed to become chronic, it can lead to pedal osteitis which is a thinning and demineralization of the coffin bone. Foot injuries can also result in keratomas which are tumors arising in the horn-producing cells of the hoof wall, usually in the toe region and sometimes in the sole. When the keratoma becomes large enough to cause lameness, it is usually surgically removed.

Disease as a cause of lameness

Arthritis, or what is commonly referred to as degenerative joint disease (DJD), takes a number of forms. It is the end result of various injurious processes. The disease usually begins with an inflamed joint capsule and can progress into erosion of the cartilage and fusion of the joint. Degenerative joint diseases affect both young and older horses. Stiffness and diminished range of motion are the hallmarks of lameness associated with arthritis. Infectious or septic arthritis occurs when bacteria from the blood stream invade the joints destroying cartilage and causing irreversible damage.

Bone spavin is the name given to arthritis of the hock joint. It is an occupational hazard in horses that are ridden at a hard gallop such as jumpers, race horses, and hunters. Typically bone spavin disappears as a horse warms up and reappears when the horse cools down and is known

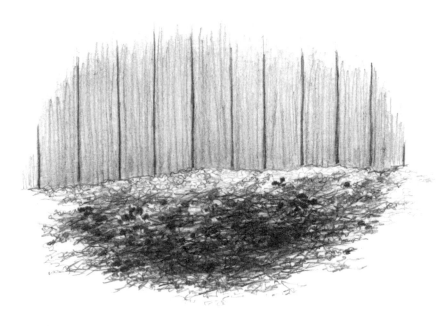

Hoof abscesses

Hoof abscesses are extremely painful causes of lameness. When bacteria invades the hoof capsule, the inflammation causes pressure that must be relieved by your veterinarian. Avoid this cause of lameness by keeping your horse's pen clean of standing water and manure.

as a " cold" lameness. Osselets is an arthritis of the fetlock joint and may affect one or both front feet. In the initial stages stretching or tearing of the fetlock joint capsule is accompanied by signs of acute serous arthritis. As the arthritis advances, pain and swelling occur along with new bone growth causing the horse to take short, choppy strides and plant weight on the outside edge of the hoof.

Shoulder joint arthritis is another common form of arthritis. It often occurs after a fracture caused by being kicked by another horse, running into a stationary object, or by a hard fall. Osteochondrosis of the shoulder joint in growing horses may cause sufficient joint injury to lead to a degenerative arthritis.

Azoturia or tying-up syndrome are degrees of a condition known as exertional myopathy which occurs when horses that have a heavy workload have a break from activity, but continue to consume a high-carbohydrate diet. When an accumulation of glycogen builds up in the muscle as a result of lack of activity, lactic acid is released and damages skeletal muscle causing it to release muscle enzymes and myoglobin. When the myoglobin is excreted in the urine, it blocks the nephrons, causing kidney failure. The resultant lack of kidney function causes the horse to become anxious, sweat profusely and develop a rapid pulse. The major muscles then stiffen causing the horse to stagger and wobble and eventually to collapse.

Upon the first indication of azoturia or tying-up, all activity should stop and the horse should be given absolute rest with no physical movement at all--not even returning to the stall. The horse should be spoken to calmly and covered with a blanket. A veterinarian should be called to provide medical relief to prevent further kidney damage and aid recovery.

> ## Note
> ### Stiff and sore joints
>
> Arthritis is common in older horses and people alike. While a variety of medications exist to control pain, one of the more important things you can do is to keep your horse active through turn-out and weekly exercise.

Nutritional imbalances, especially in growing horses can lead to lameness caused by developmental orthopedic diseases which include a group of related conditions such as osteochondrosis, osteochondritis, dissecans, physeal dysplasia, and wobbler syndrome among others. In each case, a breakdown occurs in the mechanism by which cartilage is converted to bone. The resultant abnormal cartilage is prone to fracture, fissure and break into small fragments that can enter the joint causing lameness. Although some horses appear to have a genetic predisposition for developing DOD, external factors include a too-high energy diet accompanied by insufficient calcium or phosphorus in the diet resulting in inadequate mineralization of bone. Also, a deficiency of microminerals such as copper and zinc, can result in defective cartilage formation.

Research shows that the most common feeding practices responsible for nutritional imbalances leading to lameness include feeding too much grain, feeding alfalfa hay without adding phosphorus to the ration, feeding a grass hay and grain mix inadequate in calcium, phosphorus, and protein, adding excess vitamins and minerals to the ration. Laminitis, also known as founder, is a diet-related disease that commonly occurs when the horse consumes excess quantities of carbohydrates that alter the bacterial balance in the cecum, indirectly leading to the release of lactic acid and endotoxins. The lactic acid and endotoxins cause the large digital arteries to the feet to dilate, increasing the blood flow while causing intense constriction of the small capillaries that nourish the laminae in the horse's foot. Deprived of oxygen, the laminae swell, the swelling damages the sensitive tissue in the foot, and unless the situation is relieved the inner structure of the feet may die causing a characteristic stance in which the two front feet are placed out front to take weight off the horse's toes.

The horse develops a high fever and chills with sweating, diarrhea, a fast pulse and rapid heavy breathing. The feet become hot and painful, and if all four feet are involved the horse may draw its feet up under its belly and lie down. Although death from founder is uncommon, it can occur. In cases of severe founder, the hoof may slough off.

Excess consumption of either too much grain or over-eating of lush, fast-growing summer pasture grasses causes most cases of founder. It can also occur during the winter if the horse consumes too much legume hay.

Another cause of laminitis is the drinking of large amounts of cold water by an over-heated, hard working horse before being cooled down properly. Laminitis becomes chronic when lameness and pain continue for more than two days. Chronic laminitis can cause permanent damage to the foot when the coffin bone becomes detached from the hoof wall and rotates so that it drops down. In severe case it can penetrate the sole of the foot.

Other complications of laminitis include white line disease, thrush, separations of the hoof at the coronary band or sole, and complete loss of the hoof. Acute laminitis is a medical emergency and a veterinarian should be called immediately to prevent the possibility of permanent lameness and disability.

The foot of the horse and lameness

According to research most causes of lameness are found in the foot of the horse. Domesticated horses living in paddocks and stables with limited opportunity to toughen their feet are susceptible to a number of foot problems.

Foot wounds that are contaminated and allow foreign bodies, bacteria, yeast, fungus, dirt, and debris to gain entrance to sensitive parts of the foot lead to abscesses and infections that cause lameness, especially if they are not noticed and treated promptly.

Thrush is a painful bacterial infection in the frog. Characterized by a putrid black discharge along with poor growth and degeneration of the horn, it is caused by lack of proper foot care resulting in a buildup of mud, manure and debris that prevents air getting to the frog.

Canker is a chronic infection of the horn tissues of the foot that begins at the frog and progresses into the sole and sometimes the hoof wall. It is caused by a lack of foot care, and is usually the result of the horse standing in mud or bedding that is soaked in urine and feces. The appearance is similar to thrush, but it involves the sole as well as the frog.

Improper or neglected hoof trimming often contributes to lameness when a horse has or develops contracted heels or sheared heels. Usually corrective trimming and shoeing will prevent further lameness.

Quittor is another foot disease caused by a deep-seated infection of the cartilages of the coffin bone. Infected material is discharged via a sinus tract that opens at or above the coronet. Injuries such as being struck by another foot near the lateral cartilages and penetrating injuries of the sole lead to quittor.

Whiteline disease also known as seedy toe is caused when bacteria, yeast or fungus invades the foot and works its way up to the white line to the coronary band. Loss of horn creates a hollow space between the hoof wall and the sole that eventually is filled with cheesy material and debris.

This disease seldom occurs in barefoot horses on pasture, but occurs with horses that are kept in wet stalls or exposed to frequent wet-to-dry episodes such as walking in wet grass or being washed down on a frequent basis.

Hoof wall cracks are another cause of lameness, although some hoof cracks do not cause the horse to go lame depending on the location and depth of the crack. Once a crack is noticed, care should be taken to prevent the crack from lengthening and deepening.

Deep cracks are susceptible to infection and since new horn has to grow out from the coronary band to repair the crack, steps need to be taken to clean, stabilize, and either do corrective shoeing or repair the crack using prosthetic material.

Limb deformities and lameness

Limb deformities are usually present at birth, although some limb

212

deformities are the result of injury, especially to the joints during the first weeks of life. Congenital limb deformities are caused by abnormal limb positions in the uterus, nutritional imbalances in the mare, neonatal hypothyroidism or unequal growth between two sides of a long bone. Many normal foals have some degree of limb crookedness that straightens out by the time they become yearlings. Others need veterinarian treatment to correct the problem. Angular limb deformities include knock-knees, bow-legs, bucked or sprung knees, calf knees, benched or popped knees. Early recognition and treatment are important to prevent permanent damage. Treatment is usually based on x-rays and physical examination. Sometimes stall rest and therapeutic exercise are enough to correct the problem. Other cases may require splints, casts, braces or surgery. Treatment before three months of age works best in the prevention of future problems. Flexural limb deformities tend to affect young horses from birth to 18 months of age. They occur most often in the fetlock joint, coffin joint and knee joint and involves a shortening of either the deep, the superficial, or both digital flexor tendons. The cause is unknown, but one theory is that rapid growth of long bones is not matched by the growth of the tendons, causing the joint to be pulled into flexion. When the deformity is severe or progressing in spite of treatment, surgery is advised to divide the inferior check ligament thereby allowing the flexor tendon to lengthen. In some cases ligaments may be cut in advanced cases. In all cases, a veterinarian should be involved in diagnosing and treating the problem.

Preventing lameness

Horses are remarkably strong and adaptable creatures and any lameness in a horse in their native habitat is usually the result of an injury caused by rough terrain or interaction with other horses. Because of the circumstances of domestication and use of the modern horse, coupled with the design of their bodies, the domesticated horse is highly susceptible to lameness. The selective breeding of horses for speed, endurance, jumping, and a variety of activities has led, in some cases, to changes in leg and foot structure that also make them more prone to lameness.

As a horse owner, preventing lameness in your horse is well worth the effort and will pay off handsomely. Beginning with your daily once over, you can keep your horse healthy, athletically fit, and functioning on all four legs and hoofs, while helping to prevent lameness: While doing your daily once-over check for lumps, bumps, swellings or hot spots, especially around the backs of pasterns, lower legs, and tendon areas. This will help you catch any sign of lameness before it has a chance to progress.

Observe your horse carefully after riding or exercising to determine if the horse is moving in a comfortable and smooth fashion. If not, examine the frog and sole of the foot for bruises or foreign objects and pick the hoof if necessary to see the clean structure. Checking for increased digital pulse and/or increased heat in the foot area are important for catching hoof diseases such as laminitis and injuries in their earliest stages.

Remember that your farrier and your veterinarian are two of your horse's best friends when it comes to actively preventing lameness. Appointments with your farrier on a regular basis will enable you to make sure your horse's hoofs are properly trimmed and balanced, as well as properly shod to meet the work demands of the horse.

Your farrier will also note any signs of developing problems with the feet and lower limbs of the horse and make suggestions for correcting or treating such conditions. If you elect to trim and care for your horse's hoofs, make sure that you trim and rasp the bearing surfaces evenly so that the foot is level. Make sure you don't over trim the heels, thereby putting a strain on the sesamoids that might produce lameness. Remember that the best job of trimming a hoof preserves the angle that is normal for the horse, not one that corresponds to a picture-perfect ideal in a magazine or other source.

If corrective trimming and shoeing are necessary for your horse, the best results will come from cooperative efforts of your farrier and veterinarian. Most orthopedic diseases of horses such as laminitis, sand cracks, flat feet, sole bruises, tendonitis, sidebones and other diseases and conditions are best treated by the services of a veterinarian who can diagnose the extent of the problem and prescribe medications or other therapies, plus the services of a farrier to make sure the feet of the horse are kept in the best possible condition.

Diet and lameness

Feeding your horse a nutritious, well-balanced diet will help prevent many of the diseases and conditions related to lameness. One goal of a well-balanced diet should be to prevent obesity in your horse since obese horses are more susceptible to laminitis and metabolic syndrome that lead to serious cases of lameness. An appropriately balanced diet is essential for normal growth and healthy appearance of your horse's hoofs and musculoskeletal system no matter what age the horse is.

A balanced ration will provide adequate amounts of calcium, biotin and the essential amino acid DL-methionine. High protein, and heavily concentrated diets that increase the horse's weight without appropriate amounts of exercise should be avoided. Mineral imbalances from over supplementation also create bone problems and can lead to damage and disease in the musculoskeletal system.

Environment and lameness

Make sure that the areas where your horse lives and works are free of holes that a horse might step into thereby breaking or spraining a leg. Keep pieces of wire, nails, broken fence boards, pieces of sharp metal, machines, and other objects that your horse might run into or that might impale or injure your horse away from horse activities.

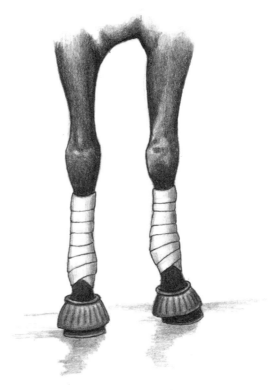

Do not let your horse stand in muck, dirty and/or wet bedding, stagnant water, mud, or other elements that are destructive to hoof, limb and general health. Change bedding frequently, muck out stalls on a daily basis and provide good drainage in pastures and paddocks and other places where water and mud contribute to unhealthy conditions not only for a horse's hoofs, but also provide a

Hoof and leg protection

Depending on both the sport and the conformation of your horse, an investment in hoof and leg protective boots and wraps can help you avoid lameness due to injury.

215

breeding place for insects such as mosquitoes. Avoid wet-to-dry-to wet episodes and keep trails and arenas as dry and free from obstacles such as large tree branches, rocks and other debris.

Use secure latches on all stable and barn doors, as well as gates and other outlets that might allow a horse to escape and endanger itself by getting onto a road or into other unsafe places.

A key part of good horsemanship is making sure that your horse has a certain level of physical comfort at all times. Using fly repellents and barn misters to keep disease-carrying flies and other insects off your horses is important in preventing conditions that could lead to lameness.

Having a scheduled deworming program is effective in controlling internal parasites that can sap your horse's strength and lead to general debility thereby making your horse more susceptible to diseases and accidents that affect limb and hoof integrity.

When riding and exercising your horse, always use good judgment. Never push a horse beyond its limits when it comes to strenuous exercise. Condition your horse gradually, and if any signs of lameness occur, rest your horse appropriately and take into consideration the horse's over-all health and stamina

Take time for adequate warm-up and cool-down periods each time you exercise your horse, and be consistent with your exercise program. Don't ride the horse strenuously one day a week and then have it stand idle the other six days.

Make sure your tack fits and is used properly. Groom your horse on a regular basis to make sure that no burrs or foreign objects create sores or painful conditions. When you climb into the saddle, stay light and balanced and don't pull all your weight against the saddle horn.

Preventing lameness should be part of your daily action plan. Being proactive and making sure that your horse stays healthy and well conditioned, while avoiding obvious threats to its limbs and feet will help ensure a pleasant, vital, and active life for both you and your horse.

Symptoms

A horse that is lame not only suffers physically and mentally, but also cannot do the work that helps maintain physical health and the sense of well being that the horse needs for a satisfactory existence. Usually, signs of lameness are perfectly obvious. The horse has a decided limp, or the horse holds one hoof off the ground and refuses to move. A lame horse may shift its weight restlessly from one foot to another or stand with its legs splayed out widely or tucked in under its body. Lame horses often don't turn circles smoothly and cannot run as far or as fast as sound horses.

When a lame horse moves, it may put more weight on the good leg than the bad leg. This causes the head to bob up and down. Watching the shoulders and hips, it's possible to see the good limb sink a little more than the sore limb because the good limb is accepting the weight of the body.

Horses that are lame because of hoof problems withdraw their painful hoof when it is squeezed or tapped with a hoof tester. Pus may be draining from an abscess that occurs within the hoof. Hoof abscesses travel upward to drain above the hoof wall at the coronet band and the blood vessels traveling to the hoof may have a bounding pulse.

Horses that are lame because of joint problems often have heat and swelling in the lame joint. Comparing the lame leg with a sound leg reveals the difference. Horses that become lame due to ligament and tendon problems often withdraw their leg if the ligament or tendon is pinched.

Lame horses often don't lift their hoofs off the ground because lifting requires joints to bend, which causes pain. These horses take short steps and may drag the toe rather than swing it upward in a normal arc.

Sometimes lameness is so subtle that the rider doesn't realize the horse is lame until a savvy observer notes a slight break in the gait or uneven hoof prints on the trail.

Since lameness can be the result of infections, degenerative and metabolic diseases, developmental conditions, and mechanical malfunctions, it may be impossible for a layman to discover the cause.

In some cases, your farrier can discover the cause of lameness and treat the problem, especially if the problem originates in the horse's foot. In other cases, it may take tests and diagnostic imaging as well as an examination by your veterinarian to discover the location and the root cause so that treatment can begin.

Diagnosis

Because lameness has many causes and the consequences of either a misdiagnosis or the wrong treatment can have devastating results for the horse, few horse owners are capable of making a definitive diagnosis of lameness in a horse. Lameness is a dynamic rather than a static event and needs to be examined under a variety of conditions to fully assess the horse's capabilities since a horse may not show the same grade of lameness under different circumstances.

The degree of lameness may vary depending on the ease or difficulty of movement, the stage of the movement or exercise, and the cause of the lameness. A horse that is walking around in a pasture may not appear to be lame, but, with a rider on it's back, may show significant lameness when urged into a trot or canter. Difficulty of terrain or different kinds of surfaces may impact the grade of lameness. A horse may show no evidence of lameness on a soft, smooth surface, but show a high degree of lameness on rough, hard terrain.

The horse needs to be observed carefully to see if the lameness worsens, stays the same, or improves under different conditions and with varying degrees of exercise. The evaluation process and comprehensive lameness examination requires patience by the horse owner and veterinarian. Cases of lameness may take several days to investigate and are even more difficult to evaluate once the lameness becomes chronic.

Another consideration for the veterinarian is whether the apparent lameness might indicate a neurological disease caused by spinal cord damage, especially if it is mild. Horses with neurologic disease often move and carry themselves abnormally causing painful orthopedic conditions as the horse attempts to compensate.

Neurological diseases such as wobbler syndrome and equine protozoal myeloencephalitis, trauma, and other diseases and conditions can cause severe neurological deficits that result in performance problems and lameness.

Horses, particularly those with chronic problems, may develop compensatory gait abnormalities to deal with the primary problem making diagnosis more difficult. This may complicate the lameness evaluation and possibly its treatment. Therefore, it is important to have both the lameness and the indications of any neurological problems evaluated as soon as they are recognized.

A systematic approach to diagnosing lameness

Prior to a veterinarian's examination to diagnose the causes of lameness, the horse should be off any pain medications for at least 24 hours. This includes Bute or Banamine, and similar medications.

A veterinarian will begin the diagnosis by taking a medical history of the horse and asking the owner about any activities or conditions that might have caused the lameness. Next the veterinarian will carefully

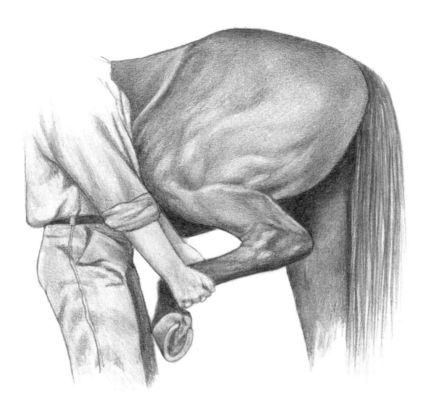

The lameness exam

An experienced horse person can easily detect lameness, but it takes a skilled veterinarian to isolate the cause and provide proper treatment.

examine the feet of the horse since nearly 90% of lameness occurs in the foot. The veterinarian will also evaluate the trimming of the hoofs, the shoeing, and may remove the horse's shoes to more carefully observe all areas of the foot.

A physical examination of the horse using palpation and manipulation of muscles, joints, bones, and tendons, joint flexion tests, and application of hoof testers will help reveal evidence of injury or stress. Part of the evaluation includes the veterinarian holding each of the horse's limbs in a flexed position, then releasing the leg. The physical examination will also appraise conformation, weight-bearing, and balance.

An evaluation of the horse in motion with particular attention paid to any deviations in gait, failure to use all four feet in sync, unnatural shifting of weight from one limb to another, head bobbing, stiffness. As the horse trots away, the veterinarian watches for signs of pain, weight shifting, shortening of stride, and irregular hoof placement.

Some veterinarians now use a Lameness Locator with sensors that monitor and record the horse's torso movement while the horse is trotting. The recorded information is then transferred to a computer or mobile device and compared against databases recorded from the movement of healthy horses and other lame horses. The computer is then able to diagnose whether or not the horse is lame.

A neurologic examination should be part of the workup since conditions such as wobblers syndrome and equine protozoal myeloencephalitis, as well as trauma and other diseases can masquerade as lameness.

Note
Showtime?

Horses that appear lame will be dismissed from the show ring at any reputable horse show. Showing or riding a lame horse can cause additional damage to the weakend joint, tendon or structure.

Blood tests to detect drugs that may camouflage lameness or that might contribute to the lameness along with X-rays to identify damage or changes in bony structures aids the veterinarian in making a correct diagnosis.

The veterinarian will also use analgesic techniques, including diagnostic regional nerve and joint blocks, to identify the location of the injury or stress that is causing the lameness. Working from the foot up, the veterinarian temporarily deadens sensation in specific parts of the limb, one joint at a time, until the lameness disappears. This procedure isolates the area of pain causing the lameness and also helps determine whether the condition is treatable.

Ultrasonography, nuclear scintigraphy (bone scan), or magnetic resonance imaging to look for soft-tissue problems involving tendons, ligaments, joint surfaces, and muscle tissue. Computer tomography (CT) may be used for both tissue and bone problems.

Samples of blood, joint fluid, and tissue are taken for examination to determine if infection or inflammation are present. These tests usually require laboratory evaluation before results are available.

In some cases, one or two of these steps in the examination of lameness may allow the veterinarian to make a diagnose and determine treatment. In other cases, all of these factors will need to be considered and additional steps taken based on the over-all condition of the horse, the severity of the lameness, and the horse owner's plans for the horse.

A thorough lameness workup with the development of related rehabilitations regimens can be complicated and time-consuming. Owners should make sure they understand what is causing the lameness, the prognosis for recovery, and the medications, exercises, therapies and other requirements to restore the lame horse to its best possible condition.

The horse owner should follow the veterinarian's instructions and be willing to comply with requests for follow-up exams. In most cases, the horse will need rest during treatment and possibly for some time afterward.

How veterinarians grade horse lameness

Because each horse has individual characteristics, evaluating lameness can be challenging. The American Association of Equine Practitioners has developed a lameness scale that ranges from zero to five, with zero being no perceptible lameness, and five being extremely lame:

1. Lameness not perceptible under any circumstances
2. Lameness is difficult to observe and is not consistently apparent, regardless of circumstances (e.g., weight carrying, circling, inclines, hard surfaces, etc.)
3. Lameness is difficult to observe at a walk or when trotting in a straight line, but consistently apparent under certain circumstances (e.g., weight carrying, circling, inclines, hard surfaces, etc.)
4. Lameness is consistently observable at a trot under all circumstances
5. Lameness is obvious at a walk
6. Lameness produces minimal weight-bearing in motion and/or at rest or a complete inability to move

Treatment

Most horse owners turn to stall rest at the first sign of lameness in their horses, and in some cases, it may be the most appropriate method of treatment. However, any lameness that lasts for a length of time should be diagnosed and treated by a veterinarian.

Treatment will vary depending on the condition diagnosed, but at a minimum usually includes rest, appropriate medication and other supportive therapies for fast, effective healing. In general, it helps to reduce your horse's weight and amount of exercise, and have your horse stand on soft, even flooring.

Currently, veterinarians have many different treatments for lameness available including acupuncture and sensory nerve stimulation to treat pain involved in lameness, along with hydrotherapy, shockwave and stem cell treatments, use of platelet rich plasma and bone marrow aspirate to treat various kinds of lameness. None of these are magic cures, nor can they replace a proper rehabilitation program, but they can potentially accelerate the healing process. More importantly, these treatments may promote better-quality healing and therefore provide the best prognosis for long-term soundness.

Arthroscopic surgery is gaining in importance as newer and better ways are developed to make use of this method of surgery for both diagnostic and therapeutic purposes. Arthroscopy is commonly used to help diagnose joint disease, especially injury to soft tissue structures that will not show up with traditional radiography such as meniscal or cruciate injuries in the stifle.

Treatment for horse lameness is most successful when it addresses the cause of the lameness and takes steps to improve the horse's environment, diet, work load and other factors that lead to lameness.

Conclusion

Horse legs evolved for swiftness and explosive power. Your horse's long limbs are useful for escape or defense in a natural setting, but can be fragile and prone to injury. Virtually all horses will show lameness at one time or another, and your ability to recognize and care for lameness is important for your horse's health.

In this chapter, you learned about your horse's basic leg and foot anatomy. Understanding the anatomy helps you recognize why lameness occurs, and also how best to detect lameness. Your veterinarian uses knowledge of anatomy to perform a lameness exam, isolating each joint and tendon to determine the source of the pain.

You have learned about the most typical causes of lameness. This is extremely helpful as your knowledge of the causes can help you understand how to prevent lameness, another important section of this chapter.

If you attend horse shows or horse events, you will often hear com-

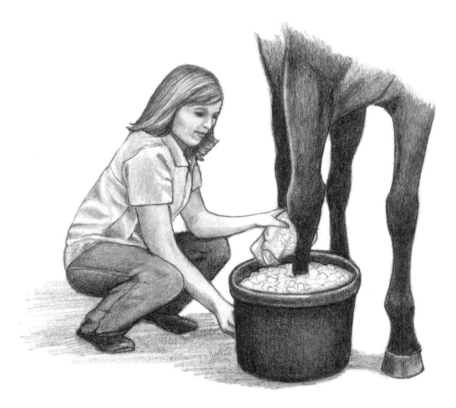

Treatment of lameness

Depending on the diagnosis, you may be required to perform daily activities to help relieve the pain associated with lameness. Along with any advised stall rest, your efforts will result in quick and proper healing of the injury.

ments from the audience such as - "That horse looks a little off. I think he has a front left lameness." Horse people love to observe and diagnose lameness, but in reality it is not so simple. Finding the source of the pain, making a diagnosis and devising a treatment plan should be left to the veterinarian. Nonetheless, this chapter has taught you how to isolate the limb that may be the cause of lameness.

The treatments of lameness are as varied as the causes, but most of them rely on stall rest for sometimes a lengthy period to allow slow mending tendons or ligaments to heal. Some dramatic lamenesses result from infections within the foot. These cases of lameness can normally be relieved by your veterinarian with a simple procedure that takes a few minutes. The important lesson is to get your veterinarian involved early so that you can follow a sound plan based on an educated diagnosis to treat the cause of your horse's lameness.

Top-5 takeaways

1. Lameness is pain in one or more limbs that affects the movement of your horse. Virtually all horses suffer lameness from time to time.

2. Your horse's legs and feet are designed for walking up to 20 miles per day in search of food, and for an occasional explosive sprint to avoid predators. The strain and stress imposed by horse riding requires special care to prevent lameness, or to treat lameness should it occur.

3. Good conformation reduces lameness, poor conformation increases lameness. Purchase or breed for a horse with good conformation, including large and symmetrical hoofs.

4. Recognizing that your horse is lame is relatively easy. Diagnosing the leg and joint or cause of the lameness generally requires the expertise of a veterinarian.

5. In most cases, lameness requires a period of stall rest. Working or riding a lame horse can exacerbate the injury, and lead to a longer and more expensive recovery.

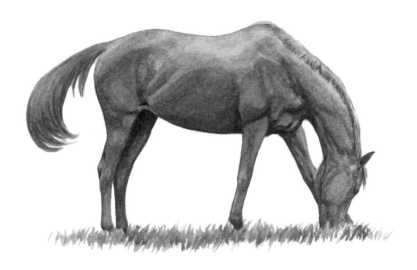

Chapter 9 Nutrition

Introduction

In the wild, horses consume a wide variety of grasses, shrubs, and foliage. They find mineral rich soils that they consume as well as the sources of fresh, ideally running water. In captivity, horses diets are often restricted to hay and feed supplements. Hay is a great source of nutrition for our horses, and is the foundation of any feeding program. Unfortunately, hay varies in quality and nutritional content, and may not provide the proper nutrients in the amounts required for your horse's health.

In this chapter, you will learn how to feed your horse a balanced and nutritious diet. You will be surprised to learn that most of the fancy and expensive food supplements are not required for horse health except in cases of disease. In general, good quality hay and an adequate supply of minerals is sufficient for the typical horse.

Senior horses may require additional consideration to cope with nutritional requirements. Older horses may have problems properly chewing their food, or may suffer from metabolic conditions related to age.

Younger horses or horses in training may need more protein and calcium to assure proper bone and muscle growth. You will need to adjust your feeding program in both cases to make sure that the proper nutrition is provided.

Horses in the wild spend the majority of their time browsing for food. The horse's digestive system is designed for this method of consumption that is characterized by a continuous stream of a variety of feeds throughout the day.

The carnivore method of feeding, that we use to feed our dogs and cats, is based on large meals at infrequent times (once or twice a day). Horse health and mental state are improved as we move from a carnivore method of feeding to an herbivore method of feeding. This means small frequent meals throughout the day. This may be best accomplished with a properly designed free-choice feeding system that is outlined in this chapter.

The natural horse diet

The horse's digestive system and its nutritional requirements have not changed since it was domesticated thousands of years ago. A horse's digestive system is long and complex with a relatively small stomach. Digestion begins as soon as the food enters the mouth and the food then passes in a steady stream into stomach and the intestines. Rapid ingestion of feed causes the stomach to empty rapidly before the stomach enzymes can act upon the entire meal. This interferes with total digestion and proper use of nutrients.

When the horse became domesticated, it became dependent upon its owner for its feed, usually of the hay and grain readily available and at the convenience of the owner. This meant that the horse was given a large amount of feed usually twice a day. Unfortunately, the horse's digestive system has not had time to evolve to meet these new demands of larger less frequent feedings, and, as a result, horses have a number of problems related to feeding and their digestive system. Since a horse is unable to vomit or belch, consuming too much feed too rapidly can have disastrous consequences. Because the horse's colon bends back upon itself numerous times, it leads to greater utilization of the roughage in the horse's feed, but can also cause digestive problems when a horse is not fed properly.

One of the first natural needs of the horse that we need to recognize is the fact that horses need small amounts of feed frequently throughout the day to maintain a healthy digestive system. In addition, they need a supply of clean, fresh water, minerals and micro-nutrients to keep their digestive system functioning properly.

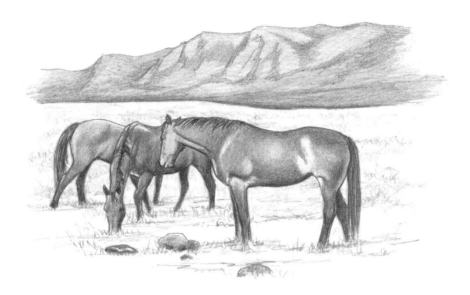

Horse digestive system

In nature, the horse forages over large areas in search of food consisting of grasses, forbs, bushes and mineral deposits. The domesticated horse has feeding requirements driven by digestive capabilities resulting from this natural diet.

Feeding a better and more natural diet

A diet of high quality hay or grass will provide all of the energy and protein that a non-working horse requires. Remember that there are big differences between legume hay such as alfalfa and clover and grass-type hays such as Bermuda and Timothy. Equine nutritionists recommend feeding your horse as frequently throughout the day as possible. When feeding hay, weigh it to make sure you are giving your horse the correct amount for its needs and, if possible, place the hay in several small piles either at ground level or slightly above to allow your horse to assume a better position when eating in a more natural grazing manner. Place the hay on low feeders or on rubber mats or other protective surfaces if you are afraid your horse will ingest sand or dirt.

Choose your hay wisely since all hay is not the same. Good hay is leafy as opposed to having too many stems. It will be a light green color as opposed to brown or dark. It will have a fresh, sweet smell with no moldy or musty odor and will contain a minimum of weeds and debris. A variety of hays and grasses from different sources should be fed to help prevent nutritional deficiencies as a result of hay grown in deficient soil

If your horse's work level makes feeding grain necessary, feed a natural grain diet instead of heavily processed feeds. Supplementing your horses diet with oats, corn or barley, or a combination of mixed grains works well for most horse owners. Pay attention to well-researched advances in feed science, and be sure to purchase quality grain and feed according to the needs of your particular horse.

In addition to its regular feed, consider giving your horse a tree branch or a branch from an edible shrub occasionally to help keep its teeth in working order. In nature horses browsed on shrubs and tree limbs which were tough enough to smooth rough edges on teeth and keep the jaws moving in a natural pattern.

> ## Note
> ### Probiotics
>
> A horse's digestive tract relies on a variety of bacteria to do a large share of the digestive process. Sometimes changes in feed or the use of antibiotics may upset the balance of these beneficial "bugs." You can easily administer probiotics packaged for use in horses to help replenish the natural digestive bacteria.

As a horse owner, educate yourself about available feeds and use your knowledge to choose wisely for your horse. If a horse is in training or is ridden frequently, you may want to supplement the diet with grain. Remember to read and compare feed tags when buying grain and supplements for your horse, and consult with your veterinarian before making any abrupt changes in your horse's diet.

To keep the horse's digestive system working properly, every horse needs a supply of fresh, clean water. In nature, horses wade into streams and ponds, giving their hoofs an occasional moisturizing bath. Because of the horse's diet, access to water, and natural walking and running that a horse enjoyed in the wild state, the horse's hoofs usually stayed healthy.

In addition to forage and water, horses should have access to a free-choice salt and a trace mineral product formulated for horses.

Although it may be impossible to imitate nature completely, by taking a few cues from the way horses satisfied their dietary needs in the wild and integrating them into the way you feed and water your equine, you can lay the foundation for a healthier, more energetic animal.

Nutritional requirements

The horse's digestive system and its nutritional requirements have not changed since it was domesticated thousands of years ago. The horse's digestive system continues to obtain maximum nutritional benefit from a diet of high fiber and low energy grasses and hay. A nutritionally complete diet for a horse will contain water, energy, fiber, protein, carbohydrates, fatty acids, minerals, and vitamins.

Paramount to meeting feeding requirements of horses is the fact that horses need to be fed small amounts frequently to maintain a healthy digestive system. With a small stomach, a small intestine that is 70 feet long, and a large intestine that adds another 25 feet to the digestive system, the horse needs to continually eat small amounts of feed. This feed is ideally digested over a rather long period of time as it passes through the intestines where the nutrients are extracted. A horse's relatively small stomach can hold only one to four gallons of food at a time, but the food moves into the gut track very quickly so the horse feels hungry again about an hour after eating. Infrequent feeding of large amounts also creates an imbalance in intestinal bacteria, resulting in stomach disturbances, diarrhea, and colic. It can also contribute to gastric ulcer disease, estimated to afflict 60% to 90% of mature horses.

Ulcers occur when stomach tissue is damaged by digestive acids. Because a horse is meant to graze on an almost continual basis, his stomach constantly produces digestive acid for the breakdown of food. When there is food in the stomach, the acid is properly absorbed and neutralized. Allowing your horse free access to pasture or grass hay, while cutting down on grain and concentrated processed feeds, lowers his risk of developing ulcer disease. It also reestablishes a more natural feeding pattern and wakes up his foraging instinct.

> ## Note
> ### How much to feed your horse
>
> Most horses need between 1-½ to 2-½ % of their body weight each day in forage. There are many variations in the nutritional requirements that depend on the animal, such as age, breeding status, temperament, existing diseases or conditions. Horses that are worked daily or compete may also need grain to provide enough nutrition for the additional work

The second natural dietary need that needs to be addressed is the amount of feed a horse needs to eat to maintain healthy body weight given the work load of the horse. Most nutritional experts agree that a horse should consume at least 1.5 to 2 pounds of quality hay, grass, and grain for every 100 pounds of body weight. Horses with heavy work loads and pregnant and lactating mares need to consume up to 3 pounds of dry matter for every 100 pounds of body weight.

A third important natural dietary need of the horse involves the need for a variety of plants in its diet to make sure it gets the necessary nutrients, as well as the necessary amount of chewing and roughage to keep all components of the digestive system in top working order. A horse will nibble eagerly on all kinds of vegetable matter including tree branches and other hefty plants with thicker stems and branches in addition to grasses and hay. Eating a variety of vegetation helps wear down the horse's teeth which are continually growing. In the wild, horses did not need to have their teeth rasped, but instead fed in such a way that the growth of its teeth were naturally kept under control.

A fourth factor to consider in feeding a horse is the fact that wild horses foraged for feed on the ground for the most part, occasionally reaching up for tree branches or into bushes and chewing on coarser vegetation. Most feeders in barns and stalls force a horse to eat with the neck extended and the head raised instead of lowered. With the neck extended and the head up, the horse cannot properly chew its feed, the amount of saliva decreases, tooth wear is uneven and the possibility of choke or obstruction increases. In addition, fine debris and grass particles bombard the horse's face and neck and can lead to respiratory problems as the horse inhales the falling dust and debris.

A fifth factor to consider in meeting the natural dietary needs of horses is that in the wild, horses ate very little if any grain except for natural grasses and plants that had gone to seed. Since plant seeds ripen in the fall, the timing was good for the horse since it could gain extra weight to carry it through the winter months. Modern, domesticated horses are often fed too much grain considering their workload and body condition. This leads not only to obesity, but also to additional health problems.

If your horse's work level makes feeding grain necessary, feed a natural grain diet instead of heavily processed feeds. Supplementing your horses diet with oats, corn or barley, or a combination of mixed grains works well for most horse owners. Pay attention to well-researched advances in feed science, and be sure to purchase quality grain and feed according to the needs of your particular horse.

A sixth item of key importance in meeting the horse's natural dietary needs is the importance of minerals which are crucial for normal functioning of the horse's body. Minerals affect energy production, fluid balance, growth, bone formation, and rate of healing. Mineral imbalances can cause a variety of skin, hoof and intestinal problems, as well as stress intolerance and lowered immune reserves. Horses should have access to a free-choice salt and trace mineral product formulated for horses. Most horses instinctively limit themselves to what their bodies need when it comes to salt and trace minerals. In some cases, your veterinarian may recommend supplementing your horse's diet with

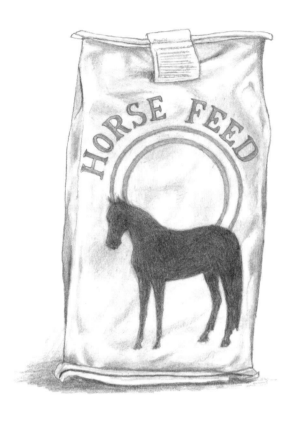

What is a healthy diet?

Proteins, carbohydrates, fats, minerals, vitamins - If your horse cannot procur his own feed, you will need to make sure that the diet is balanced and complete.

other minerals and vitamins. These should be given directly to make sure that the horse gets the right amount at the right time.

The seventh important factor to consider in the nutritional needs of your horse relates to furnishing plenty of clean, fresh, palatable water. For the most part, horses in the wild tended to live near streams, lakes or other natural water sources. Most horses like to submerge their entire muzzle into water if given the chance. Not only do they snort and play with the water, but doing this helps clean out the nostrils and provides a refreshing moment especially on warm or hot days. Unfortunately, many horse watering bowls or troughs do not allow this kind of activity because they are too shallow or not at the correct height.

When providing water for your horse, follow nature as closely as possible with low shallow troughs or bowls that allow the horse to drink closer to the ground. Always make sure that troughs or bowls are clean and algae-free and contain plenty of fresh, clean, palatable water. Occasionally allow the trough or water bowl to overflow to give the horse's hoofs an occasional moisturizing bath especially in warm dry weather. Don't over do letting your horse stand in water, however, because too many wet-dry episodes can lead to drying, cracking hoofs.

> ## Note
> ### Electrolytes and water
>
> During hot weather, and especially when exercising or competing with your horse in hot weather, his natural salts and potassium levels may become reduced. This depletion may contribute to heat stroke, or anhydrosis - a conditions that can be deadly. Adding electrolytes, either commercial or homemade, to your horse's water or grain helps combat these serious conditions.

Although it may be impossible to imitate nature completely, by taking a few cues from the way horses satisfied their dietary needs in the wild and integrating them into the way you feed and water your equine, you can lay the foundation for a healthier, more energetic animal.

Body scoring

Prior to 1983, no universal way to assess and communicate body condition was available. Then, along came Dr. Don Henneke, a professor of animal sciences and director of equine science at Tarleton State University, Working with colleagues, Dr. Henneke created a universal scale to assess a horse's body weight. This condition scoring system is based on visual appraisal and palpable fat cover on six areas of the horse's body.

Because "fitness" is subjective, equine health care professionals utilize a "Body Condition Scoring" system to measure horses in relative terms. The horse's physical condition is rated on visual appraisal and palpation or "feel" of six key conformation points including the amount of flesh or fat covering along the neck, the withers, down the crease of the back, at the tailhead, on the ribs and behind the shoulder at the girth.

According to the AAEP and veterinarians, for most horses, body condition scores in the moderate to moderately fleshy range of 5 and 6 are ideal. A common suggestion is to keep your horse in a physical condition where you can feel the divisions between the ribs, but not be able to see them.

Here is the way the Henneke Body Condition Scoring System describes the horse on the 1-9 scale:

1. Poor: Animal extremely emaciated; spinous processes, ribs, tailhead, tuber coxae (hip joints), and ischia (lower pelvic bones) projecting prominently; bone structure of withers, shoulders and neck easily noticeable; no fatty tissue can be felt.

2. Very Thin: Animal emaciated; slight fat covering over base of spinous processes; transverse processes of lumbar vertebrae feel rounded; spinous processes, ribs, tailhead, tuber coxae (hip joints) and ischia (lower pelvic bones) prominent; withers, shoulders and neck structure faintly discernible.

3. Thin: Fat buildup about halfway on spinous processes; transverse processes cannot be felt; slight fat cover over ribs; spinous processes and ribs easily discernible; tailhead prominent, but individual vertebrae cannot be identified visually; tuber coxae (hip joints) appear rounded but easily discernible; tuber ischia (lower pelvic bones) not distinguishable; withers, shoulders and neck accentuated.

4. Moderately Thin: Slight ridge along back; faint outline of ribs discernible; tailhead prominence depends on conformation, fat can be felt around it; tuber coxae (hips joints) not discernible; withers, shoulders, and neck not obviously thin.

5. Moderate: Back is flat (no crease or ridge); ribs not visually distinguishable but easily felt; fat around tailhead beginning to feel spongy; withers appear rounded over spinous processes; shoulders and neck blend smoothly into body.

6. Moderately Fleshy: May have slight crease down back; fat over ribs spongy; fat around tailhead soft; fat beginning to be deposited along the side of withers, behind shoulders, and along sides of neck.

7. Fleshy: May have crease down back; individual ribs can be felt, but noticeable filling between ribs with fat; fat around tailhead soft; fat deposited along withers, behind shoulders, and along neck.

8. Fat: Crease down back; difficult to feel ribs; fat around tailhead very soft; area along withers filled with fat; area behind shoulder filled with fat; noticeable thickening of neck; fat deposited along inner thighs.

9. Extremely Fat: Obvious crease down back; patchy fat appearing over ribs; bulging fat around tailhead, along withers, behind shoulders, and along neck; fat along inner thighs may rub together; flank filled with fat.

The job or workload of a particular horse also has a bearing on what weight is appropriate for maximum performance. Polo, race and endurance horses might be perfectly fit with body condition scores of 4 or moderately thin, while a body condition score of 7, fleshy, may be required for success in the show ring. However, by feeding a horse to a level of 8, the limits of good health are being pushed. Horses with scores of 8 and 9 are definite candidates for a weight reduction plan.

Forage and grain

Most horse owners recognize the value of forage as the main part of their equine's diet. Down through history, horses have foraged for the plants and grasses that are rich in nutrients and developed a sixth sense about which plants not to eat.

Over the years, horses developed a specialized digestive system based on their natural feeding pattern of continuous ingestion of grass and other forage.

Many different types of hay are acceptable in horse feeding programs. Local availability often influences the popularity of a particular variety of hay in a geographical area. For example, coastal Bermuda grass hay is popular in the southern United States where it is well adapted, but it is rarely fed in the northern U.S. where it is hard to grow.

In Kentucky, the most popular hay choices for horses are alfalfa, timothy, orchard grass and alfalfa-grass mixes. Somewhat less popular, but still common are red clover, fescue, and Bermuda grass.

Several factors should be considered when deciding what type of forage to feed. Although purity and cleanliness of the forage is important, the nutrient value and the type of horse being fed need to be considered.

Pastures are a rich source of nutrients for your horse. As most horse owners know, quality forage, whether it is hay or pasture, should be the foundation of any horse's feeding program. Good quality pasture can provide much of the nutrition a horse needs.

Another important fact about pastures is that they also provide an economical source of forage. The cost of pasture as a feed is estimated to be about one-tenth the cost of hay.

The ability of pasture to supply the feed requirements of your horse

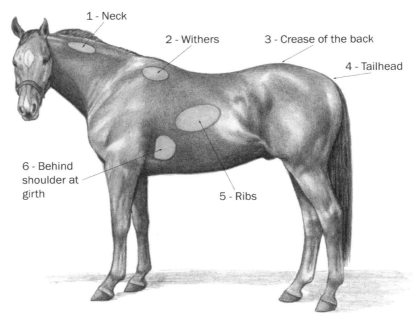

1 - Neck
2 - Withers
3 - Crease of the back
4 - Tailhead
6 - Behind shoulder at girth
5 - Ribs

Areas to inspect for body scoring

Horses gain weight and deposit fat into specific areas of the body depending on the available diet. Closely monitoring these areas can help you determine that the diet meets, but does not exceed the horse's caloric requirements.

will depend on several factors including the species of grass and hay growing in the pasture - Legumes are higher in protein and digestible energy (calories) and lower in fibre than grasses. Therefore, a pasture with a higher proportion of legumes, such as alfalfa or clover, will possess a higher nutritional value compared to an all-grass pasture.

The plant's stage of maturity also affects its value as forage - Pasture forages are high in nutritional value when actively growing and become lower in nutritional value with maturity. The more immature the plant, the more nutritious and palatable; however, the smaller the plant, the less feed it provides.

The season of the year often determines the nutrient value of forage - Spring grass contains the highest levels of protein and lowest levels of fiber. As the grazing season progresses into summer and fall, a reduction in growth and an increase in maturity of the forage leads to lower nutritional value.

The horse's physiological state determines its nutritional needs - In many cases, good quality pasture can meet the nutritional needs of most adult pleasure horses, along with water, salt and trace mineral supplementation. Even growing two-year old horses can get all they need from good quality pasture.

Weanlings, yearlings, pregnant and lactating mares and horses in hard work, however, may need more than an all-pasture diet. These groups of horses have higher nutritional requirements and will likely require grain feeding as well as grazing.

Taking representative samples of the forage growing in your pasture at different times of the year and sending them to a laboratory for chemical analysis is the most accurate way to help you determine the overall feeding value of your pasture. A hay analysis gives horse owners the level of crude protein, total digestible nutrients, calcium, phosphorus, magnesium and potassium in the hay, and can be a valuable investment.

When purchasing hay for your horse, a number of factors come into play. As grazing animals, research has shown that horses do best when their feeding patterns follow a natural grazing pattern. The length of time the horse spends foraging for food and the amount of feed eaten at one time are important things to consider.

Compared to other non-ruminant animals, the horse has a relatively small stomach, normal-sized small intestine and a large hind gut. This digestive arrangement makes the horse better suited to grazing continuously than to having one or two large meals a day.

Hay and other roughage provide nutrients and satiety for your horse. On average, a horse must consume about two percent of its body weight per day to maintain body weight and digestive health. Different ages, classes and workloads of horses require different levels of nutrients from the hay they eat.

A combination of these and other factors make choosing the right type of hay for your horse a challenge, but with a little consideration, you as a horse owner are in a position to analyze and compare and make the best choice for your particular horse.

Most horse owners are familiar with only a few types of hay, depending on the part of the country in which they live. However, a vast array of hays are commonly fed to horses in the United States, including timothy, orchard, alfalfa, coastal, oat, fescue, clover and rye, to name just a few.

A number of types of hay can help meet the nutritional needs of horses

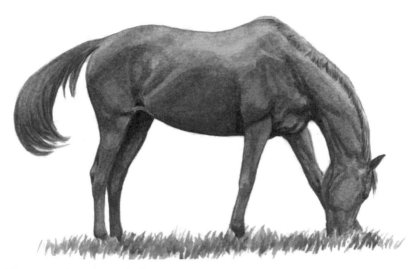

Horses love grain!

Sugary and tasty, many horse owners feed grain just because their animals
love it. Except for the high-level performance horse, most horses do not need
a grain supplement.

when fed according to the individual horse's needs and level of activity,
while some are not recommended as horse feed. Before selecting which is
most appropriate, it's important to be familiar with these common types.

Commonly fed legume hays include alfalfa and clover, with most other
hays falling into the grass family. Legume hays have a higher protein
content than grass hays, and should be fed to active, working, lactating,
young or convalescing animals that have higher nutritional needs. It can
also be used as a treat for adult animals. Most animals like the taste of
alfalfa hay, however it is too rich to use as the only daily hay for most
non-working adult animals. It should be fed in moderation, or fed as a
blend with grass or grain hays.

Alfalfa hay

Alfalfa is the predominant type of hay harvested in the U.S. About 40
percent of U.S. hay acreage, 55 percent of hay production and 60 percent
of hay value over the past five years has been alfalfa and alfalfa mixtures.
Alfalfa can be grown successfully in most areas of the U.S. It generally has

higher nutrient content, yields higher tonnage, especially in the irrigated areas of the western U.S., and brings a higher price than other types of hay.

Several characteristics of alfalfa make it an excellent hay for horses. It is highly palatable and most horses will readily consume alfalfa hay. However, because of its high palatability, intake must be restricted to keep horses from overeating and becoming colicky.

Alfalfa hay is high in energy. It has 120 percent more energy per unit in weight than oat hay. Therefore, it takes less hay to meet a horse's nutrient needs when feeding alfalfa hay. However, the high-energy content may lead to overfeeding and to a fat horse.

Alfalfa hay is high in good-quality protein. Crude protein values can be as high as 18 to 19 percent. People once thought that feeding alfalfa hay to horses caused kidney damage because of increased urination and ammonia production. We now understand, however, that excess protein in alfalfa is converted into energy compounds, and the nitrogen produced in this conversion must be eliminated as ammonia.

> ## Note
> ### Hay analysis
>
> Some hay producers routinely analyze their hay, and many provide the results to the horse owner. If you buy your hay in bulk, and your producer doesn't provide this service, you can have sampled hay analyzed yourself (ask your veterinarian for a test lab and procedures).
>
> The service provider or your veterinarian can help you understand the test results, and may recommend certain supplementation if the hay is deficient in important nutrients.

Alfalfa hay is also a good source of vitamins and minerals. If cured correctly, vitamin C content will be high. The calcium to phosphorus ratio is about 6:1 and must be considered when feeding young, growing horses.

There are generally five to eight cuttings from an alfalfa field each year when irrigated, four to five when not irrigated. The first cutting will have more weeds and grass; the second cutting is usually clean with small stems. The third cutting is good hay, and the fourth and fifth cuttings begin to have more stems and fewer leaves. As more stems are present, the quality of the hay decreases and palatability declines.

Grass hays

Grass hays have a lower protein content, and are suitable for easy keepers, and other horses that do not require the extra calories. In general, grass hays are less expensive than legume hays, but because of demand by the horse market in some areas, grass hays can be more expensive. Pricing is highly regional.

Many horse owners prefer a mix of legume and grass hays as an ideal forage for their horses. Various mixes are available in baled form, or you can buy bales of legumes and grass, and then vary the feeding. Many commercial stables will offer a choice (e.g. alfalfa in the AM and grass in the PM).

Timothy hay is one of the most popular hays fed to horses. It can be quite expensive, depending on whether it has to be shipped long distances. Timothy must be harvested in the pre- or early-bloom stage to ensure a high nutrient content.

Timothy grass is grown primarily in the northeastern portion of the United States and also in California and Nevada. Timothy is not a very drought tolerant plant and does not respond well to excessive heat. Timothy grows best in areas with abundant day length and moisture. Timothy grass hay is commonly fed to horses, as well as cattle. It is relatively high in fiber, especially when cut at a later or more mature stage.

Timothy is typically harvested two times per season, the first cutting in early summer and the second cutting in late summer or early fall. The first cutting is typically preferred for feeding to horses as it has longer and harder fiber length, as well as longer seed heads. Some first cutting is also fed to cattle. Second cutting is typically fed to cattle, but in some cases is also utilized for horses.

Timothy hay is 10% protein. It is a good source of copper and zinc and has a good balance of protein and energy.

Oat hay is an excellent feed for horses. The choice between alfalfa and oat hay depends on price per unit of energy or protein and the type of horse being fed. Depending on the area of the country in which it is grown, oat hay can be low in protein and contain only marginal calcium, phosphorus and carotene.

Oat hay is best cut when the oat seed is out of the milk stage and into the dough. This ensures a high quality product still showing some color with good carbohydrate content and sweetness in the stem. Cutting at the proper time means animals will eat the entire hay stem with little waste. Oat hay, like all grass hays, meets the nutritional needs of herbivores that need high fiber and low protein.

Clover hays

Clover hays are similar to alfalfa hays because they are legumes. Clover hay is usually mixed with grass hays. There are five kinds of clover hay: red, common white, crimson, alsike and landino. White and landino clovers are usually grown for pasture. The other three contain 14 to 16 percent crude protein.

Hay or pasture containing a large percentage of alsike clover is generally not recommended for horses because of its toxicity. The symptoms of alsike poisoning vary and susceptibility seems to depend on the area where the clover is grown and the individual horse.

Clover hay can cause "slobbers" in horses. The condition is caused by a fungus, Rhizoctonia leguminicola, commonly known as black patch that grows in clover that is not properly dried prior to baling. Slobbers is excessive salivation that generally does not hurt the horse, but is not pleasant to be around.

> ## Caution
> ### Forage quality counts
>
> Mold, dust, weeds, blister beetles, old tin cans. Take caution when buying hay and buy it from a reputable feed store or farm supplier. If you buy your hay without attention to quality, get ready for allergies, bouts of colic, diarrhea or worse. You should establish a relationship with a quality feed source that understands the nutritional requirements of your horse, and who you can trust to provide quality feed.

The most common symptom of "slobbers" is photosensitization or a reaction to light. The real problem, however, which is not so readily observed, is liver damage. When purchasing hay, it is best to make sure that it contains little or no alsike clover.

Fescue hays

Tall fescue is a hardy, popular, cool season perennial grass that can grow on a variety of soils in a variety of climates. It is grown on an estimated 35 million acres in the U.S.

Tall fescue has a high yield. It is drought resistant, resistant to overgrazing and is a high quality nutrient source.

Fescue hay can cause toxicosis in pregnant mares when they eat tall fescue that is infected with an endophyte fungus, Acremonium coenephialum . Both the mare and the foal can be affected. Before feeding fescue hay to pregnant mares, a horse owner should make sure that the hay is free of the endophyte fungus.

Bermuda grass hay

Bermuda grass hay is used mostly in the southern United States. Common Bermuda grass does not grow tall enough for hay production, but coastal Bermuda grass can be used. The same stand of grass can be cut four or five times a year. It is as nutritious as Timothy hay, and its value can be increased by growing it with a legume.

Some Bermuda hay is grown in the Imperial Valley of California, a region that provides the right conditions to grow top-quality Bermuda hay. Bermuda is a less expensive alternative to Orchard or Timothy hay for those horses that are fed grain or supplements. With less protein than alfalfa, 8% - 10%, it is an excellent source of roughage for all types of livestock. Additionally, it is a good source of vitamin A and D without an overload in protein, and it has a better balance between calcium and phosphorus.

Orchard grass hay

Orchard grass is a flat leaf, bladed, perennial, cool season, tall-growing grass. Orchard grass is high in fiber and low in protein to help support a healthy digestive tract. The leaves vary from green to bluish green depending on the maturity of the plant.

Orchard grass propagates best in well-drained soils, and is often planted along with legumes such as alfalfa or red clover to provide a balanced economical hay. Care must be taken to cut orchard grass hay at the proper stage, as older stands of orchard grass will produce course and less palatable hay.

Hays to avoid

Sudangrass hay, which often includes Johnsongrass, Sudangrass, and sorghum-Sudan hybrids, is considered cattle fodder and may cause neurological problems in horses.

Horse owners are warned not to allow horses to graze these plants as they may develop cystitis syndrome. This condition looks like colic with accompanying bloody urine and can be fatal to horses. Affected animals may show a staggering gait and urine dribbling. Pregnant mares may abort. There is no treatment for this poisoning and poor prognosis of recovery.

When choosing hay use the sight, smell and purity test: Do you see plenty of leaves as opposed to rough stems and is the hay a pale greenish brown? If the hay is mostly stems and is dark or black in color, don't buy or use it.

Does the hay have a pleasant smell? Hay should smell fresh. Moldy or too dusty hay should be avoided at all costs.

Does the hay consist of just hay or is it full of sticks, weeds, rope, foreign objects or other debris? If so, it's not worth the time or trouble and your horse's health would suffer in more ways than one.

Supplements

Scientific research in horse nutrition over the past few decades has answered many important questions regarding the need for supplements in a horse's diet. Beyond simply contributing to your horse's good health, supplements, when used appropriately, can help prevent disease and illness as well as add vim and vigor to the horse's daily activities.

In addition to water, the five main classes of nutrients that your horse needs to survive include fats, carbohydrates, protein, vitamins and minerals. In many cases, veterinarians add electrolytes to this list, especially when the horse is athletically involved or does heavy work in conditions with high temperatures and humidity.

When your horse is lacking in any of these main classes of nutrients, supplements can fill that void to keep your horse healthy and strong. In addition, when certain diseases or conditions strike, a supplement may be the ticket to healing the disease or correcting the condition.

But, which supplements are truly necessary, and which supplements may be a waste of your time, effort, and money?

Having evolved as non-ruminant, herbivore grazers that typically spent around 18 hours a day grazing pasture grasses and other plants, horses developed a rather unique digestive system.

The horse has a very small stomach that holds between 2 and 4 gallons in the average 1,000 pound horse. Because of the small stomach, the horse's small intestine, which is 50 to 70 feet long and holds around 12 gallons, does most of the work of digesting and absorbing the nutrients in the hay and other feed the horse eats.

From the small intestines most of the liquids and roughage are then passed on to the cecum where toxic substances are detoxified and where bacteria and protozoa create fermentation that helps digest most of the fiber and soluble carbohydrates and produce essential fat-soluble vitamins that are absorbed by the horse.

Keeping your horse's digestive system and work load in mind as you make decisions regarding supplements is very important.

Once the horse ingests a substance, it must go all the way through the digestive system because horses cannot regurgitate, so feeding too much of a supplement or a supplement your horse doesn't require can create problems.

Many horses need only good forage, water, and a mineral block to maintain body weight and regular activity.

When hay is of poor quality or instances when a senior horse has a hard time chewing and digesting roughage, the addition of an appropriate amount of beet pulp added to the diet in small increments may be all that is needed for a good maintenance diet.

Since carbohydrates are the main energy source in most feeds, many horses do not need additional carbohydrate supplements.

Protein

Veterinarians often recommend protein supplements for older horses, weanlings, pregnant and lactating mares, and horses with a heavy work load or high exercise level. Ordinarily, adult horses require 8 to 10% protein in their feed.

Signs of protein deficiency include reduced growth, weight loss, loss of performance, a rough hair coat, and low milk production in the case of lactating mares.

Proteins are made up of linked amino acids. They are the structural components of muscle and ligaments and are a source of energy. Horses need protein supplements when their diets lack essential amino acids such as lysine that are not normally synthesized in their bodies.

When choosing a supplement or a complete feed, protein is often listed first on the tag or label. Protein is an expensive ingredient and the manufacturer of the supplement or feed is required to give a minimum value of crude protein in the feed. Feedstuffs that contain more than 20 percent crude protein are considered to be protein supplements.

The quality of the protein is also important based on the amount of lysine it contains. Synthetic lysine is often added to make sure the feed has a sufficient amount of that amino acid.

Soybean meal with approximately 44% crude protein is the most common protein supplement. It is considered to be a high-quality source of protein with the proper ratio of dietary essential amino acids. Alfalfa hay with 17-22% crude protein is also considered to be a good source although the quality of the hay will affect the actual protein value.

Other sources of crude protein include, canola meal 40%, cottonseed meal 45%, and peanut meal 53%, although these are not as commonly used in supplements and feed for horses as soybean meal.

A number of commercial products including complete, pelleted, and sweet feeds are available that claim to incorporate a balanced nutritional source of protein for horses of different ages and activity level. In all cases, reading feed tags and contents of protein supplements is extremely important.

> ## Note
> ### Local and fresh is best
>
> When it comes to forage, ideally choose locally grown hay in bulk when it is in season. You will find the best quality and price from a local supplier, especially if you commit to purchasing a 6 month or 1 year supply.

Fats

Fats are a concentrated source of energy and are necessary in the horse's diet to absorb fat-soluble vitamins and provide linoleic acid, the essential fatty acid. Although most feeds contain less than 6% fat, this amount is adequate for the nutritional needs of many horses.

Performance horses, horses with a heavy workload, pregnant and lactating mares, and under-weight horses often need fat supplements.

The most commonly used fat supplement is vegetable oil. It can be added as a top dressing to the horse's regular feed, beginning gradually with a quarter of a cup per feeding and working up to no more than two cups a day for an average size horse. (1,000 lbs. / 454 kg.).

Rice bran is another fat supplement that is gaining popularity. Rice bran is about 20 percent fat and also supplies vitamin E and energy. Owners of performance horses use rice bran for supplementation because it helps horses maintain or gain additional weight if needed, while giving show horses a sleek and healthy appearance.

Rice bran is also palatable and easy to store and handle. Gradually adding one to two pounds to the horse's regular daily diet is usually sufficient. This amount of rice bran does not upset the balance in the horse's diet. In addition, the vitamin E is helpful in fighting the results of stress in horses that undergo strenuous exercise and changes in their environment when traveling to activities.

Don't overdo fat supplements. Since a horse does not have a gallbladder, digesting and utilizing a too much of a high fat supplement is not only difficult, but is also wasteful.

Vitamins

Although plenty of vitamin supplements are available on the market, vitamin supplementation is usually not necessary unless a low quality forage is being fed, the horse is involved in strenuous exercise, the horse is ill or recuperating from surgery, or is being fed a high grain diet.

Vitamin D is obtained from sunlight, so only horses that are kept in their stalls 24 hours a day need supplemental vitamin D. Vitamin E is found in fresh green forage. Vitamin K and B-complex vitamins are produced by microbes in the horse's intestines and vitamin C is found in fresh vegetables and fruits and is produced in the liver.

Severely stressed horses may benefit from B-complex and vitamin C supplements, and performance horses may need additional vitamin E.

Fat-soluble vitamins include vitamin A, D, E, and K, and water-soluble vitamins include C and the B-complex vitamins

Supplemental vitamins should be used with caution, especially the fat-soluble vitamins that include vitamin A, D, E, and K. These may reach toxic levels if over ingested because they are stored in the body if not needed immediately. Water-soluble vitamins include C and the B-complex vitamins and don't usually pose any problems because any excess vitamins are excreted in urine and through sweat.

Minerals and micronutrients

Mineral supplements are often required in the horse's diet since they play a vital role in the horse's health. Although horses are able to obtain a large portion of their mineral requirements from their feed, mineral availability and concentration varies with the soil content, plant species, and stage of maturity when the feed is harvested. A reputable mineral block will often provide all the minerals a horse needs.

Minerals are involved in maintenance of structural components including muscles, bones, and ligaments. They play roles as enzymatic cofactors and are involved in energy transfer in the horse's body. Minerals are also necessary to provide maximum absorption of vitamins, as well as adequate functioning of hormones and amino acids. Organic minerals supplied with a balanced diet help prevent muscle abnormalities, developmental orthopedic disease, and other health issues.

Generally, the major minerals of concern in supplementing a horse's feed are calcium, phosphorus, and in some geographical areas selenium. Ground limestone is a good source of calcium, and either monosodium or disodium phosphate are a good source of phosphorus. Dicalcium phosphate is the most common supplement used to provide both calcium and phosphorus.

Research has shown that calcium, zinc, copper and phosphorus benefit a horse's overall health and reduce cases of muscular problems. Trace mineral blocks are the most common way to meet trace mineral requirements. Organic minerals have been shown to have a positive effect on the immune system, development of cartilage in young horses, and healthy hoofs in horses of all ages.

Some horses will take to eating dirt or their stools when they have a mineral deficiency. Check with your veterinarian if this happens with your horse. Your vet can advise you about what may be missing in your horse's diet to satisfy his appetite without resorting to dirt or stool ingestion.

Electrolytes

Horses have a natural craving for salt and an adult horse will consume about one-half pound of salt a week. Lactating mares and horses in training will consume more. If a free-choice salt block is available, most horses will consume enough to meet their needs without developing salt intoxication, if sufficient water is available.

Several medical studies have shown that supplementing a horse's diet with electrolytes, when appropriate, can be very beneficial, especially when the horse is hard working and subjected to strenuous exercise while competing in racing or endurance events or in cases where the horse sweats excessively.

Electrolytes come in various formulas and usually include sodium, chloride, potassium, magnesium, calcium and other minerals often mimicking the same balance as found within cell membranes. Avoid commercial formulas with added sugar and dyes.

Adding electrolytes to the feed works much better than adding them to the water, simply because the horse may not take in enough water to make the supplementation effective or may refuse to drink it if the water tastes different.

Generally, beginning electrolyte supplementation a few days before an event and continuing for a few days after the event works well to help the horse perform at the best possible level, while not suffering from the strain of the exercise. In some cases, low doses of electrolytes may be recommended on an on-going basis.

Make sure you follow the proper dosage recommendation for your horse. If the diet you are feeding is adequate and balanced, the only electrolyte supplementation you may wish to consider is sodium and chloride (salt), since sufficient potassium and other minerals are in the horse's feed.

In all cases, your veterinarian can help you determine what supplements will work for your horse and which supplements will be a waste of time, effort and money.

Specialized supplements

Senior supplements: Specially formulated for stiffness, discomfort, weight loss, poor digestion and weak immunity, these supplements may help horses as their bodies begin to function less efficiently.

Joint, hoof and coat

Joint, hoof and coat supplements: Joint supplements are used to relieve stiffness and soreness, and are often used in competition horses. Key active ingredients are glucosamine, hyaluronic acid, and chondroitin sulfate considered to be excellent for sustaining healthy joints and supporting horses with joint problems, as well as relieving excessive inflammation in conditions such as osteoarthritis.

> ## Note
> ### Don't over supplement your horse
> It is a waste of money to supplement a horse for no medical reason. Ask your veterinarian about the needs of your particular horse prior to purchasing supplements. Except for special needs horses under the care of your veterinarian, focus your nutrition dollars on high quality forages in the proper balance and amounts and nutritionally required minerals and vitamins that are not provided by your forage.

Hoof supplement formulas usually contain biotin, methionine and other ingredients essential in the production of keratin which is necessary for healthy hoofs.

Ingredients for maintaining healthy coats are often combined with joint and hoof supplements and include the addition of Omega 3 and fatty acids in a flax seed base.

Digestive

The horse's digestive systems are surprisingly delicate with performance horses often suffering from ulcers and other horses being hard keepers whose digestive systems lack the balance to maintain health and prevent digestive complications such as colic. In some cases, a veterinarian will recommend special feed or a digestive supplement to protect the horse's digestive system.

Probiotics and prebiotics along with amino acids claim to promote regeneration and repair of cells that line the intestines as well as help your horse's system utilize the base diet and gain full benefit of any nutritional supplements.

All the rest

Respiratory supplements are formulated to address chronic or seasonal respiratory problems by soothing and supporting the horse's irritated airways. Horses with allergies, heaves, stable cough and other respiratory conditions may benefit from these supplements.

Muscle products are designed to help build up muscle protein, delay the onset of fatigue, and prevent muscle breakdown during and after heavy workouts or competitions.

When a horse has anhydrosis, a failure to sweat properly, supplements for the condition are sometimes necessary. This condition is most often found with horses that live in hot, humid climates. The formulas usually include ascorbic acid, niacin, L-tyrosine and cobalt proteinate which have been found to be effective in university field tests.

Yeast cultures are thought to supercharge the microorganisms in the hindgut that break down fiber and reduce the build-up of acid. They may also be helpful in balancing the chemical compounds found in the horse's gut and help with the digestion and absorption of nutrients by the body. In lactating mares, the ingestion of yeast cultures helps pass on potent nutrients to foals enabling them to be healthier and grow at a better rate.

Herbal products have become very popular both for people and animals. The key element in herbal treatments is supposed to be a restoration of harmony and balance in the body. Unfortunately, not all companies offer full disclosure of ingredients, fillers, strength, etc. of their herbal compounds. In most cases, herbals are medicinal and should be administered only with the advice of a qualified health practitioner or veterinarian. Many herbs are banned by equine sport governing bodies. Be sure to check with the appropriate association before giving herbal supplements to competition horses.

Formulated for the "anxious, spooky, worried" horse, calming supplements claim to help the horse relax and focus on the work at hand. Formulas often include thiamine (vitamin B1) and magnesium which are essential for the stability and normal function of the cell membranes of excitable tissues such as nerve and muscle.

Many supplements are available in the market place. By feeding your horse a balanced diet, you can minimize the need for supplements. Instead, healthy treats such as carrots and apples can be part of your horse's diet, along with a little molasses, some cod liver oil, a good salt lick and when horses need it, some beet pulp that has been thoroughly soaked before feeding to add energy and protein to the diet. Remember that not all supplements are created equal. Read labels and dosage information carefully, and always check with your veterinarian before adding supplements to your horse's diet.

Water

With a large body, the horse needs clean, fresh, palatable water at least several times a day, if not free choice all the time. In a horse, dehydration is often not recognized until 5 percent or more body weight is lost and when a loss of 6 to 8 percent occurs, a horse can be in serious trouble.

A horse's body contains 62 to 68 percent water with a 10 percent variation being accounted for by differences in age, amount of body fat and muscle mass, and the amount of exercise during any given period.

Water is essential for all metabolic activities and for a number of vital physiological processes including utilization and digestion of nutrients, regulation of body temperature, muscle contraction strength, joint lubrication, and waste elimination.

The typical horse weighing 1,000 to 1,200 pounds needs 8 to 10 gallons of water each day just for maintenance, and during strenuous exercise in hot, humid weather when the horse is sweating a great deal, it will need 2 to 3 times more.

A lactating mare producing 3 gallons of milk a day needs at least 75 percent more water per day and during hot weather that need can increase significantly.

Many horses are given access to water only a couple of times a day. Although horses can adapt to this practice, it is not always best for their health and well-being. A horse going without water for a number of hours will begin to become dehydrated and the functioning of its body will begin to decline.

When temperatures are cold and drinking water temperatures approach freezing, a horse's water intake will usually decrease drastically. This is not good, and, in fact can lead to problems such as impaction colic.

According to research, horses prefer water that ranges between 45 and 65 degrees Fahrenheit, and will drink more water if it is in the proper temperature range. Ask yourself, "Do you like to drink hot water on a hot day, or icy water when the temperature is around freezing?" Neither does your horse!

During cold weather, care should be taken to make sure that water is warmed to a drinkable temperature. This is extremely important for older horses or horses that have chronic illnesses. An automatic heating element can be used in many cases to keep water at a drinkable temperature

> ## Note
> ### Make your own electrolyte mix
> Electrolyte mixes basically consist of sodium chloride (table salt), and potassium chloride. A combination of these salts provide theessential electrolyte components of potassium, chloride and sodium. A basic recipe for an electrolyte mix includes 1 ounce of table salt and 1 ounce of lite salt (contains potassium chloride). Add this amount to a 5 gallon bucket of water for daily consumption. Added sugars and flavorings are not necessary nor desirable.

Water availability should never be left to chance. Frozen water troughs, fouled water buckets, broken automatic systems, natural rivers or streams that are polluted or contaminated, wrong-size water buckets, and water troughs filled with algae all lead to horses not getting enough fresh, clean, palatable water, and in the worst case scenario becoming dehydrated and ill because of lack of water.

Fortunately, there are several effective ways for providing water for your horse and thereby making sure it he maintains the proper fluid balance in his body for maximum health and efficiency.

Buckets that are automatically filled several times a day, other automatic waterers, water troughs that are systematically cleaned and refilled regularly, heated water buckets or troughs used during cold weather, and many other options are available for the horse owner who wants to ensure the health of the horse by always having an accessible water supply available.

In addition to making sure your horse always has access to plenty of fresh, clean, palatable water, you should recognize when your horse is becoming dehydrated and its fluid balances need attention.

Signs of dehydration are weakness, depression, sunken eyeballs, dry mucous membranes, slowed capillary refill time, and increased heart rate.

Quite often dehydration is caused by prolonged strenuous exercise in hot, humid weather. An overworked horse that has lost too many fluids through sweat can become a victim of heat exertion which can be fatal if not addressed quickly.

In worst case scenarios where both temperature and humidity are high, the horse's systems can shut down quickly when the horse sweats, losing precious water and upsetting the electrolyte balance.

Being proactive by providing water frequently and supplementing electrolytes before, during, and after strenuous exercise or endurance riding is the best way to prevent serious dehydration.

According to research, a horse loses 75 mg. of sodium chloride and 30 mg. of potassium chloride in 25 pounds of sweat.

In addition to strenuous exercise, certain diseases and conditions can affect your horse's fluid maintenance. Cases of diarrhea, fever, acute gastric dilation, intestinal obstruction and peritonitis can lead to dehydration and electrolyte imbalance. In some cases, intravenous solutions may be necessary if the horse's systems are near shut-down because of dehydration.

When you are shipping or transporting your horse, care must be taken to make sure your horse remains hydrated. Research shows that trips over 12 hours duration create great stress on a horse. Making sure that your horse has water at least every four hours and some wet hay available during transport helps keep your horse properly hydrated and helps ensure the health and well-being of the horse.

Special needs

Many horses have special needs when it comes to nutrition. Horses that are younger or older, those have nutrition-related diseases such as laminitis or insulin resistance, those that are too fat or those that have been neglected to the point of starvation have different requirements for the nutrients that promote good health.

No matter what age your horse is, what condition it is in or what its requirements are for necessary energy to meet workload demands or special training requirements, knowing about what constitutes good nutrition and feeding your horse accordingly will allow your horse to reach his maximum potential.

Most foals get all the nutrition they need by nursing during the first

2 to 3 months of life and are commonly weaned by the age of 6 months. When a foal is a few days to 3 weeks old, it will often begin nibbling on the mare's grain and hay.

Nutritionists often recommend a creep feed ration for foals beginning around 2 months. A creep feed ration is a concentrate mix composed of processed grain specifically formulated to meet the needs of a nursing foal. A creep feed ration allows the foal to gain weight at a faster rate than a foal that continues to get all its nutrition from nursing and it helps prevent a compensatory growth spurt after weaning that greatly increases the risk of a developmental orthopedic disease

An orphan foal or a foal rejected by its mother has special dietary needs beginning with a supply of colostrum if it is not able to nurse shortly after birth. This special milk, high in fat, vitamins, minerals and protein along with immunoglobulin antibodies and other immune substances that protect the foal from neonatal diseases is extremely important

Lack of receiving the necessary colostrum is cited as the singular most important cause of neonatal infection and death during the first few weeks of life and provisions should be made for all foals to receive colostrum shortly after birth, whether from the mare or another source.

The dietary energy and water requirements of the young foal are high amounting to approximately 14 quarts per day for a newborn foal. When it is necessary to raise the foal by hand, you will need to furnish milk substitute in the correct amount with careful attention to feeding and hygiene. A good quality milk-replacer will have at least 20 percent crude protein from milk sources, at least 15 percent fat and no more than 0.2 percent crude fiber.

Once the foal reaches the age of 5 to 7 months, weaning usually takes place. Most weanlings will consume 2 to 2.3 percent of their body weight in feed per day. The daily ration should consist of a hay to grain ratio of 40 to 60 percent by weight. The weanling should also consume at least 1 pound of good-quality roughage for every 100 pounds weight.

Over-feeding can become a problem in weanlings and growing horses because of excessive weight gain and spurts of growth that may cause developmental orthopedic disease. Feeding more than 6 to 8 pounds of grain is not necessary unless hay quality is poor. The daily allotment of high-quality legume hay should be restricted to 1/2 pound per 100 pounds of weight and supplemented with good quality forage.

The average horse has reached 65 to 70 percent of its mature weight

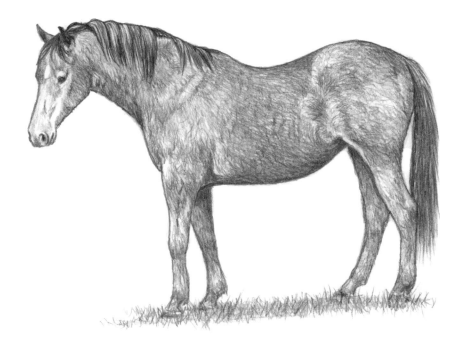

Dietary requirements must be adapted

Older horses, horse's with metabolic conditions, overweight horses - you may need to adjust your horses diet considering fairly common diseases and conditions.

by the time it is a year old. At this time, growth slows and nutritional requirements change.

Feed for yearlings should be approximately 50 percent hay and 50 percent grain by weight. One pound of grain mix concentrate per 100 pounds of weight, up to a maximum of 9 pounds should be fed. Once a young horse reaches 90 percent of its anticipated adult weight around age 2, feed can consist of all the free-choice good quality hay or pasture the horse wants to eat along with .75 to 1 pound of grain mix per 100 pounds of body weight per day.

This feed program can continue for the next several years or until the horse's dietary requirements change based on work load, exercise level or other factors.

As a horse ages, his digestive system undergoes changes and becomes less efficient. Hormonal and metabolic changes may interfere with the ability to digest, absorb and utilize essential nutrients in feed. In addition horses lose teeth and develop tongue, gum and other mouth-related problems. This creates difficulty in chewing feed properly.

The special needs of senior horses make it likely that you will need to re-evaluate your feeding program as your horse ages. Feed should be highly palatable, easy to chew and swallow and clean and dust-free to prevent possibilities of allergies and lung disease.

Some horses are known as hard keepers. No matter how much feed is available, they remain thin and even emaciated. An underweight horse with little appetite doesn't just look unhealthy, it has no energy reserves to draw on, so is easily fatigued as well as vulnerable to injury and disease.

Occasionally, horses may have or be recovering from serious conditions such as cancer, inflammatory/infiltrative bowel disease, parasitism, colitis, or surgery that have led to weight loss, and their owners are doing all they can to help the horse regain his previous condition. When feeding these horses, it is important to remember that months of minimal eating on the horse's part cannot be reversed in a few days or weeks.

Research shows that many diseases in horses have a nutritional component. While some diseases may be caused by improper feeding or inadequate nutrition, others, not directly related to nutrition, can be helped greatly when the horse's need for certain nutrients is met.

Any disease that causes a reduced appetite or overall decrease in feed intake increases the need for a higher percentage of the proper nutrients to ensure that the horse's daily nutritional needs are met.

Anemia is an example of a condition that results in a reduced appetite and reduced feed intake, yet responds to treatment when increased minerals, proteins and B vitamins are added to the diet.

Diseases that are directly related to the metabolism of certain nutrients may be inherited or common in certain breeds. Azoturia is an example of a condition that affects draft horse breeds that perform hard work during the week, are rested on the weekend without a decrease in their grain allotment, and then cramp up when back on the job on Monday morning.

Any disease that causes damage to the intestinal wall increases the need for specific nutrients for tissue repair. Colic due to gastroduodenal ulcers and enteritis are examples of a disease or condition that puts the horse's digestive system at risk and requires special nutrients both to cure and repair the damage.

Diarrhea which is involved in many diseases and conditions in horses decreases the absorption of nutrients, especially electrolytes and protein and increases the need for additional intake of these nutrients.

Laminitis is one of the most frightening diseases that relates to the diet of the horse. It occurs most often in horse breeds with high body weight, those on a high grain diet, and horses that have access to a lush green pasture.

Proper horse management is the key to preventing laminitis. By avoiding feeding excesses and keeping the horse at a reasonable weight, the horse is less susceptible to laminitis. Horses should not be turned out in lush pastures for long periods of time and should be pulled off and put in a dry lot when necessary.

> ## Note
> ### Traveling with your horse
> Some horses are very particular about their water supply and refuse to drink water if it smells or tastes different. It is important to keep your horse hydrated when traveling, so you may need to bring water from home, at least for consumption while traveling.

Insulin resistance resulting in a diabetic-like condition in horses often responds to proper dietary management of the horse. Whether insulin resistance actually becomes a significant health issue depends on the interaction between this metabolic type and the environment, specifically diet and exercise.

Insulin resistant horses may also be predisposed to allergic or exaggerated inflammatory reactions because of elevated levels of inflammatory cytokines. These problems, rather than weight issues, may be what brings the horse to the attention of the veterinarian. The worst case scenario is the acutely laminitic horse with uncontrolled insulin resistance.

For reasons that are not entirely clear, some laminitic horses are sensitive to alfalfa. This may be because some amino acids can trigger an insulin response, or it may be related to the higher starch and glucose in alfalfa hay. Horses on alfalfa that do not respond well should be switched to grass hay.

Other health problems and diseases related to nutrition include diseases that are responsive to vitamin E supplementation such as equine degenerative myeloencephalitis, and white muscle disease, and some types of hoof problems that react well to supplemental biotin and methionine.

As a horse owner, your skill in feeding your horse cannot be replaced no matter what the feeding recommendations are. Your good judgment in educating yourself about the horse's dietary requirements and knowing what works best are extremely important.

Conclusion

Most horse owners would agree that eating is their horse's favorite activity. The natural horse eats almost continuously during his wakeful hours. The food that he consumes is not particularly nutritious, and in times of drought, probably not particularly tasty, but nonetheless - horses love to eat.

Equine scientists have found that horses prefer a variable diet when given the choice. Horses also are self limiting in their food consumption if the diet is balanced and not missing specific nutritional elements. The natural horse is seldom overweight, even in times of bountiful graze.

Your challenge is to provide nutrition for your horse with these natural concepts in mind. Consider feeding at least three meals a day, and not the traditional two. Vary the feeds that you give. Perhaps a quality grass hay for one meal, and alfalfa for the next. The mixing of a grass hay and a legume hay is generally a good choice, taking advantage of the nutritional characteristics of each.

You may notice that your horse resorts to stool eating, or licking the soil from time to time. You have learned that this may signal a lack of one or more minerals or vitamins in your horse's diet. Always provide a salt block and a mineral supplement designed for horses. Talk to the county agent in your area about the hay that you feed. Ask about mineral deficiencies that may occur in hay grown in some areas of the country. This is very important if you have a pregnant mare, as the lack of certain vitamins and minerals during pregnancy can result in a miscarriage.

Don't forget to have abundant and reliable water available for your horses at all times. The horse diet requires a huge amount of water for processing. Expect your horse to drink 8 to 10 gallons a day and up to 20 gallons if working in a hot climate.

Top-5 takeaways

1. A balanced diet for your horse consists mostly of high quality forage. Depending on your sources of hay, you may wish to mix a grass hay with a legume hay (such as alfalfa) to provide variety and

reduce the chances of nutritional deficiency.

2. Most horses do not need grain or additional supplementation other than high quality forage. The exceptions to this are working horses, pregnant mares or stallions, and special needs horses (older horses or horses with a metabolic condition).

3. Fresh water, salt and trace minerals should always be available. For most horses, a combo mineral-salt block is the best choice. Also, most horses prefer troughs and buckets to automatic waterers.

4. It is best to feed more often in smaller quantities. Once-a-day feeding is not well suited to horses.

5. Feed your horse only the amount that is required to maintain a body score of 5 or 6. In general, horses are happy eating between 1.75% to 2.75% of their body weight each day. For a 1000 lb. / 453 kg. horse, this equates to 17.5 lbs. / 8 kg. to 27.5 lbs. / 12 kgs a day.

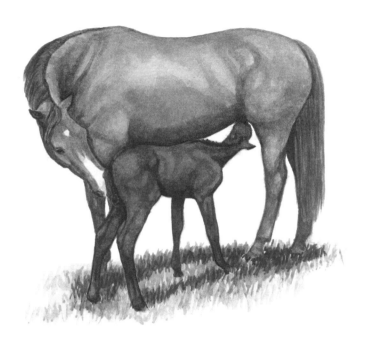

Chapter 10 Reproductive Care

Introduction

For many horse owners, the choice to breed is made for completely rational and reasonable reasons. Working ranches breed horses as replacements for the horses used to manage livestock. Competitors breed horses to leverage specific talents that are demonstrated by their breeding animals. Other horse owners simply enjoy the process and beauty of having a young horse born and raised in their care.

Unfortunately, some horse owners breed their animals in a quest for profit or to have an "experience" for themselves or their children. Others may not take adequate care of their breeding animals, resulting in unwanted pregnancies. It is not uncommon for a neighborhood stallion to escape and breed with your mare in many rural settings. In these last cases, the result is an animal that will live for up to 30 years and require lifelong care, perhaps with people that are unable or unwilling to provide the needed care.

Beyond simple care, a horse also requires a level of training that will render it safe for potential owners, farriers and veterinarians. It is truly a huge responsibility when you choose to breed your horse and any breeding should be seriously considered by the horse owner.

This chapter will help you make the decision regarding the choice to breed a horse. It will also provide you with essential information about the reproductive nature of the horse, and the information that you can use to select a proper stallion for a breeding. You will learn the veterinary process, as well as the various methods used, to obtain a healthy foal and mare.

This chapter will also covers the horse's reproductive system, and provides information about the care of the animals reproductive system, including some easily avoided diseases and conditions.

> ## Note
> ### How we use our horses
>
> Racing - 844,531 (9%)
>
> Showing - 2,718,954 (29%)
>
> Recreation - 3,906,923 (42%)
>
> Other - 1,752,439 (19%)
>
> Total - 9,222,847
>
> Other includes ranch horses, rodeo, carriage, police, polo and other uses.
>
> (Source: "National Economic Impact of the U.S. Horse Industry", American Horse Council, 2005)

Reproductive cycle

The ideal age to begin foaling is around four years of age. Mares are capable of continuing to breed until late in life and do not usually suffer ill effects if nutrition and condition are maintained. Generally in March, many mares begin to develop ovarian activity. This early activity may not be accompanied by ovulation, but beginning in May, with longer daylight hours, warmer temperatures, and the arrival of green grass, nearly all mares are cycling consistently, with conception rates peaking in June.

The best time for mating is determined by several factors, including the length of daylight, the daily temperature, the mare's general nutrition, the amount of rainfall, the climate, and the latitude. As increasing daylight stimulates the receptor centers in the brain to trigger reproductive hormones, these hormones begin the pattern of regular periods of estrous, also known as heat. The estrous cycle is the time period from one ovulation to the next. The average cycle is 22 days and this can vary by a few days especially at the beginning or ending of breeding season.

During estrus, the pituitary gland releases a follicle-stimulating hormone that causes egg follicles within the ovary to grow and produce increasing

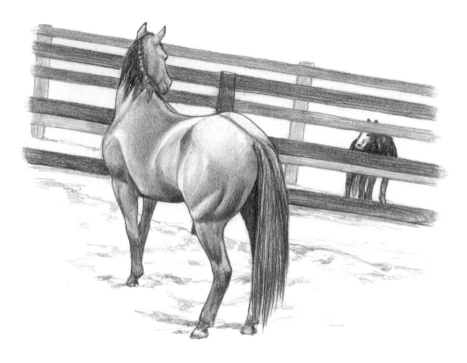

Stallion + mare = foal

Traditionally, horse breeders use live cover, having the stallion and mare copulate, for breeding. Today, breeders use technology to widen the scope of available stallions for breeding their mare.

amounts of estrogen, which prepares the reproductive tract for mating and fertilization. The increased amount of estrogen also affects the behavior of the mare. When the egg follicle approaches maturity, a second hormone is released that causes the follicle to ovulate, usually about 24 hours before the end of estrus. A normal pregnancy in horses lasts approximately 11 months or 340 days. Some mares tend to carry foals by as much as three to four weeks longer.

Breed registries and racing associations have designated January 1 as a universal date of birth for foals no matter when the foal is actually born. In racing and competitive events, a horse born in January has an athletic advantage over one born in June. For this reason, manipulation of the estrous cycle has lead to an operational breeding season beginning February 15 and ending July 15.

Regulating the estrous cycle

By exposing the mare to a longer period of daylight by using artificial light, the onset of regular estrous cycles can be hastened, making breeding possible much earlier in the year. If the breeding season is scheduled to begin February 15, artificial lighting needs to begin on December 1.

> ## Note
> ### Breeding calculator
>
> Dates, dates, dates! Breeding your mare requires knowledge of various "milestones" that will require breeder activity.
>
> We have developed a simple breeding calculator that you can use to establish a timeline for the important events on a mares breeding calendar. Access this, and other tools by visiting:
>
> https://horse-health-matters/tools

Along with the manipulation of daylight, ovarian activity is often manipulated to allow mares and stallions to remain in competition during breeding season and to facilitate the scheduling of breeding appointments. Veterinarians often administer prostaglandin or human chorionic gonadotropin, or use a Deslorelin implant to manipulate ovarian activity. Protocols have been developed in each case and a knowledgeable veterinarian can recommend what will work best for a particular mare. Altrenogests (Regu-mate®) are also used by veterinarians to shift or synchronize the time of estrus for the purposes of timing for artificial insemination. After withdrawal of this drug, a mare will predictably come into heat.

The estrous cycle produces observable changes in the mare's reproductive tract. Rectal palpitation by an experienced veterinarian or handler can detect changes in the uterus, ovaries, vagina, and cervix of the mare.

Gestation

Gestation is the period between conception and birth. A mare immunological pregnancy test is used frequently to determine if the mare is pregnant. It is 95 percent accurate, inexpensive, and convenient. Transrectal ultrasound is another option for determining pregnancy and is usually used after the 20th day, with the fetal heart becoming visible by day 30. Rectal palpitation by a skilled examiner is another way to detect pregnancy. Usually it is done as early as 20 to 30 days after service. Transrectal pal-

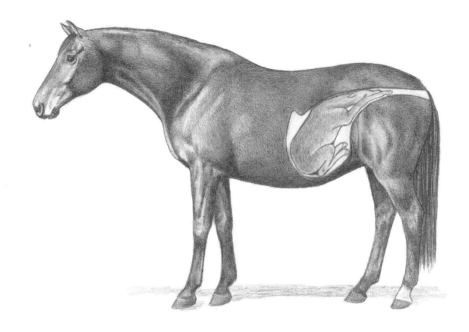

Parturition

During the final stage of pregnancy, the foal becomes positioned for a feet-first delivery. In most cases, all goes well and the delivery is quick. Have your veterinarian available "on-call," especially for new mothers.

pitation performed between days 40 and 50 is 90 percent accurate when done by a skilled examiner.

During gestation, the mare should be fed her usual ration of high-quality feed along with access to free-choice salt. During the last three months, the amount of feed should be increased approximately 15 percent since the mare will require an additional 15 percent in dietary protein and energy and twice as much calcium, phosphorus, and vitamin A. Given good care, nutrition, and a proper amount of exercise, the mare should deliver a healthy foal after approximately 340 days. Estrous usually occurs sometime between day 7 and 12 after foaling, with a second heat cycle at approximately 30 days postpartum. At this point, the mare's reproductive cycle starts over, making it possible to produce foals on a 12 month interval.

In the wild, horses usually bred during late spring, summer, and early fall to ensure that the foal was born during spring, when the weather was warming and the grass, plentiful. Foals were born fully developed and usually were able stand within 15-25 minutes of birth. They ran wild with the herd when they were one day old. This ensured that the foal would not be vulnerable to predators since a horse that could not run would be at a great risk of being killed.

The choice to breed your horse

The person who wants a horse has many options to choose from and many ways of enjoying being a part of the horse community without going through the rigors of finding the right mare and the right stallion and breeding them to produce a new foal. For those who already have a mare, some serious points need to be pondered before breeding the horse. Does the mare have valuable genetic qualities to be passed on and is she in good physical health, fertile and able to withstand the rigors of carrying a pregnancy to term? In addition, the owner or breeder should be very clear about the purpose of having a new foal. Does a market exist for the foal if the owner cannot keep the foal for its entire life, and what is the anticipated economic benefit, if any, to the owner of the new foal? Foals bred without a potential market may be sold at a loss, abandoned, or sold for slaughter as horse meat.

For the person who doesn't have a horse, one of the best ways to find out if you truly enjoy horseback riding and caring for horses is to take riding lessons. The person providing the lessons usually has several horses suited to different riding purposes and skill levels and in some cases you may be able to partially pay for the lessons by mucking out stalls which will be an added dividend since you will gain experience in horse care. If you know some horse owners, you might be able to "borrow" a horse from someone who is willing to lend you the horse. Often these horses will be semi-retired but still need some light riding activity for exercise. Sometimes busy horse owners don't have the time to give their horse needed attention, but don't want to sell the horse.

One way to enjoy the pleasure of horse activities is through leasing a horse. Often neighbors and other horse owners in your community have extra horses that, while they want to keep them, need exercise and daily care, and leasing them to a responsible person helps keep the horse healthy and active. Leasing a horse works out especially well for people who think they might want to buy a horse, but can't afford it; for those with growing children who are horse enthusiasts, but, because of growth

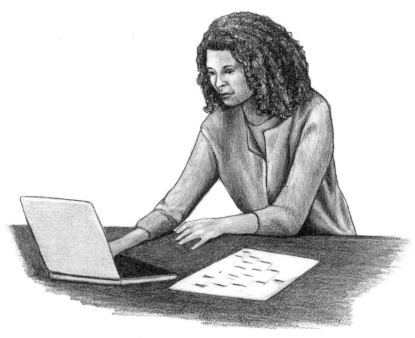

Building a better horse

Horse breeders spend hours researching possible matches for their mare. An honest appraisal of conformation and genetic qualities desired should guide the selection.

and changing interests, might want to be able to change horses; or for those who do not want the responsibilities of having a horse permanently

If you are convinced that you do want a horse for the long term, check with horse rescues and horse re-homing organizations. Rescues throughout the world are filled beyond capacity with horses of all ages, breeds, and capabilities. A little research will bring you many excellent choices and often the cost of adopting a horse from a horse rescue or re-homing organization is minimal, plus the horses come to you after having their shots, dewormings, and other health issues addressed.

Mare

A mare is a female equine over the age of three, and a filly is a female equine age three and younger. However, in Thoroughbred horse racing, a mare is defined as a female horse more than four years old. A brood mare is a mare used specifically for breeding, and a horse's female parent, a mare, is known as its dam. Careful attention to the health of the mare should be a priority before breeding takes place, during the pregnancy, and following parturition. Good nutrition, including necessary feed supplements, adequate exercise, and attention to physical condition are all important. Making sure the mare is parasite-free and up-to-date on vaccinations is also important for the ongoing health of the mare and the well-being of the newborn foal.

The mare's reproductive system

The mare's reproductive system is composed of the ovaries, fallopian tubes, uterus, vagina and vulva. The fallopian tubes carry the eggs into the uterus. This process takes five to six days. When the egg encounters a viable sperm within 12 hours the egg is fertilized and begins to grow into an embryo. The newly fertilized embryo arrives in the uterus, finally implanting in the body of the uterus at approximately the 16th day of gestation. In addition to producing eggs, the ovaries also produce the sex hormones that prepare the reproductive tract for mating, fertilization, and pregnancy.

Careful attention should be paid to the mare's reproductive health and good preparations should be made before breeding takes place. Selection of a suitable stallion, completing all arrangements for transporting the mare to the breeding farm, and having a pre-breeding physical examination to check for any problems that might interfere with fertility or breeding should be done well before the actual breeding season arrives. Mares over 15 years of age are more likely to have infertility problems. Since nutritional deficiencies, dental problems, diseases such as laminitis and Cushing's disease are more common in older mares, great care should be taken to check for any chronic problems that might keep the mare from carrying a foal to term.

Preparation for breeding

Most stallion owners require a health certificate and other health information before they will allow their stallion to breed a mare, so consideration needs to be given to obtaining the needed paperwork, especially if the mare is being taken across state lines where a health certificate showing a recent Coggin's test must accompany the horse. Your veterinarian can provide you with needed documents and requirements after the breed-

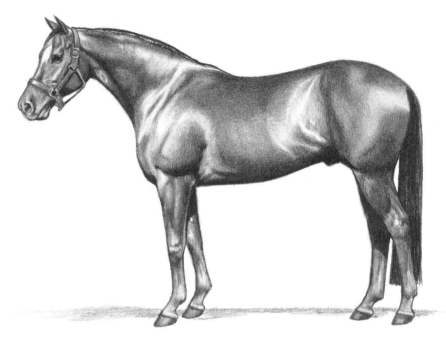

Stallion selection

Select the stallion that best reflects your ideal view of a horse, including conformation, temperament and excellent health. Consider using less known stallions to enhance overall genetic diversity.

ing soundness test. A diet that provides all the nutrients and minerals should be fed ahead of time since the effects of nutrition on fertility can be pronounced in some horses. Mares being bred should have a median body score since horses that are too fat or are too thin have a difficult time conceiving and carrying a foal to term.

Stallion

The age when a stallion reaches sexual maturity and begins to produce sperm varies from 1 to 2 years with an average of 16 months. Few stallions are ready to be used at stud before 2 years of age. At 36 months, most stallions reach their full reproductive capacity. Two important considerations in the selection of a stallion are the stallion's genetic background and his temperament.

Although there are no guarantees, it is wise to chose a stallion with a known genetic background along with a mild temperament since a foal inherits the genetic patterns of the parents and often has the same general temperament.

Preparing and managing the stallion

Management of breeding stallions usually breaks down into two basic styles: natural or confinement/isolation management. Sometimes both styles are used depending on the time of year. Natural management essentially allows a stallion to run in a pasture with a herd of mares. Proponents of natural management say that mares are more likely to become pregnant in a natural herd setting.

Some managers make a compromise between the natural and confined types of management by providing stallions with daily turn-out time in a field where they can see, smell and hear other horses. When they are stabled, bars or grills between stalls allow them to look out and see other animals.

Breeding methods

The three basic methods for breeding horses are: pasture breeding, hand breeding, and artificial insemination. Pasture breeding consists of the stallion being put out with mares in a large natural setting and allowing nature to take its course. Hand breeding allows direct management of the breeding process and provides the opportunity to select breeding individuals for complementary characteristics. It is safer and injuries to the mare or stallion are less likely to occur. The risk of sexually transmitted disease is lessened and fertility problems can be readily identified early enough to allow time to achieve pregnancy during the season. Hand breeding is also known as "live-cover breeding."

Artificial insemination became popular among horse owners during the late 1900s when the use of cooled semen proved to be successful and ways to successfully freeze semen were developed. With same-day or over-night transportation readily available in many areas, semen collected from stallions around the world can be used to impregnate mares wherever properly timed connections can be worked out. Artificial insemination has several advantages over live cover and the conception rate is usually as good or better. Advantages of artificial insemination include the fact that the mare and stallion do not have physical contact with each other, thereby reducing breeding accidents, and the chance of spreading sexually

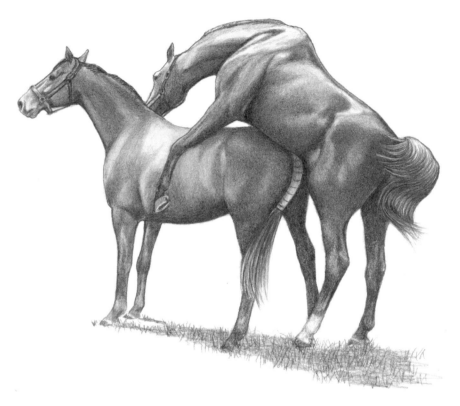

Live cover

Traditionally, horse breeders use live cover, having the stallion and mare copulate, for breeding. Today, wise breeders use technology to widen the scope of available stallions for breeding their mare.

transmitted diseases decreases. In addition, artificial insemination allows more mares to be bred from one stallion, plus, it allows mares or stallions with health issues such as sore hocks to continue to breed. Frozen semen may be stored and used to breed mares after a stallion is dead or incapacitated.

In addition to artificial insemination, several advanced reproductive technologies are now available, including Gamete Intra Fallopian Tube transfer, embryo transfer, egg transfer, and cloning. These advanced technologies are rather expensive and are rarely used by the regular horse owner.

271

Pregnancy

The gestation period for a mare from conception to foaling averages 340 days with a range of 320 to 370 days, and mares have been known to deliver healthy foals after 399 days. Foals born before 320 days are considered premature foals, and if the foal is born before 300 days, it will usually be too young to survive. When a mare fails to show heat at 18 to 22 days after service, it is often because of pregnancy. A skilled examiner can diagnose pregnancy using transrectal palpation between days 40 to 50 with 95 percent accuracy.

> ## Note
> ### Cost considerations
>
> The cost to breed and raise a horse to the age of three, broken to ride, ranges from $??? to $???. Given these costs, and the cost to purchase a horse, it is a rare case when breeding makes financial sense.
>
> Scan the QR code to learn more.

The mare immunological pregnancy test (MIP) is frequently used because it is accurate, inexpensive and convenient to use. The test is based on detecting elevated levels of equine chorionic gonadotropin in the mare's serum between days 40 and 120 of gestation. The test is 95 percent accurate. In addition transrectal ultrasound is often used to determine pregnancy, especially if the mare has a history of twins or double ovulation. In this case it is used between days 12 and 15 in order to effectively manage pregnancy reduction to a single foal. The fetal heartbeat of the foal is visible on ultrasound by day 30. Tests on plasma progesterone levels and milk progesterone levels in lactating mares are useful as early as the 16th day of gestation since they are sensitive to elevations and are 90 percent accurate.

The stages of gestation

The first 100 days of a mare's pregnancy produce few noticeable physical changes in the mare's body. During this time the mare's uterus is changing shape with the uterine horn becoming firm and tubular and the cervix becoming firm and contracted. The uterine wall becomes thinner at the site of the implanted embryo.

The mare's appetite increases and she may exhibit some moodiness. As the mare enters the mid stage of her pregnancy many veterinarians recommend a second pregnancy test because nearly one-third of mares "slip" or lose their pregnancy during the early days without the owner's knowledge. At around 150 days gestation, the foal weighs approximately two pounds and the extremities are fully formed. By 180 days, the foal will weigh nearly ten pounds and will be growing whiskers and eyelids that are capable of blinking.

By 250 days gestation, the mare shows noticeable abdominal weight gain and the foal begins gaining as much as a pound a day. The foals lungs are developing and its body is getting ready for life in the outside world as it approaches day 300 of gestation. At this time, the mare's udder distends slightly and begins producing a sticky yellow discharge that will turn to milk about two weeks prior to the foal's birth.

The mare's abdomen grows heavier and her vulva relaxes and lengthens as time for foaling draws closer. By day 315, the mare's owner should be prepared for foaling and the mare should be observed closely on a daily basis. Within one week of foaling, the foal drops and settles lower in the mare's abdomen. Her hind end relaxes and appears lower in proximity to her tail. The croup softens and the mare often shows evidence that she wants to be by herself. The mare may appear agitated and colicky and may walk restlessly. She may bite at her sides or lay down repeatedly and sweating may be obvious. This often means she is feeling contractions prior to giving birth.

Nutritional needs of gestating mares

A pregnant mare's nutrient requirements are slightly higher because she is maintaining not only her bodily needs but also is supplying nutrients to a growing

Warning
Selenium deficiency

In some areas of the country, particularly in the Western United States, selenium levels in feed are below the mare's requirements. Equine abortions are related to selenium deficiency, so consult with your veterinarian about selenium levels, and follow recommendations for supplementation if required.

fetus. During the last 90 days of pregnancy, fetal growth will increase the mare's need for energy. This means increasing the daily allotment of grain by a few pounds per day for mares weighing in the 1,000 pound to 1,200 pound range.

Daily crude protein requirements increase about a third of a pound when mares are in late gestation. Calcium and phosphorus requirements also increase during late gestation. A mare requires approximately 10 grams more calcium and phosphorus than when in an open state. As with protein, these amounts typically are met when increasing the amount of grain mix for energy purposes.

According to veterinarians, the major vitamin concern during late gestation is vitamin A. Most commercially prepared grain mixes have sufficient levels of added vitamin A to meet the mare's increased requirements adequately. Still, some brood mare managers feed a vitamin premix to guard against questionable vitamin levels.

Parturition

Pregnancies in mares are variable in length; therefore, it is important to be prepared for foaling in plenty of time. When the mare begins to show signs of beginning the birth process, it is important to watch carefully for any warning signs or irregularities that could endanger the foal or possibly the mare. The signs that foaling is imminent are noticeable as early as 6 weeks before foaling when the mare's teats and udder begin to swell and enlarge. Later the croup muscles around the tail dock and vulva of the mare begin to relax. As the mare's udder begins to fill with milk, waxing, the leaking or streaming of colostrum, forms on the teats. This usually happens 2 to 3 days prior to parturition.

The mare often becomes agitated and restless and may show colic symptoms by biting or kicking at sides, laying down, then getting up repeatedly and she may begin to sweat. Where possible, the mare may also isolate herself from other horses. Thick white milk containing colostrum usually appears 8 to 12 hours prior to foaling. This colostrum should be collected and frozen to give to the foal later.

The foaling location

Owners of domesticated horses usually make special preparations for foaling either in an appropriate sheltered place in a pasture, in a foaling stall, or in a secure place with room for the mare and any attendants necessary at foaling time. The foaling area should be clean, draft-free, warm, and dry. If foaling is to take place in a pasture, an area that other horses cannot get into should be chosen. A small, grassy paddock usually works well. Some breeders prefer having the mare in a confined area such as a

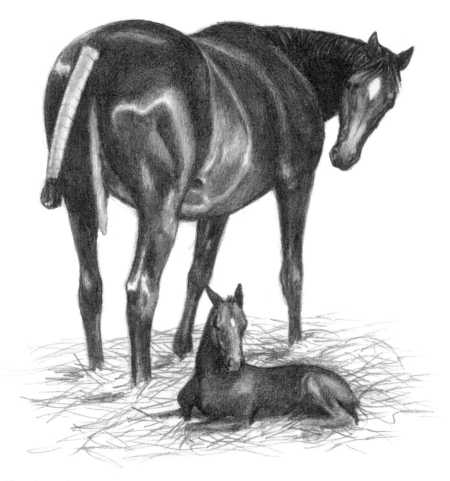

Postpartum care
Starting from birth, begin your relationship with the new foal with a focus on health and wellbeing.

box stall. If a box stall is chosen, it should be large enough for the mare to lie down and for any attendants to move safely about as necessary. The stall should be sturdily constructed, free of any sharp edges, and have good ventilation. The stall floor should be covered with several inches of clean straw , and bedding should be changed on a daily basis to maintain a clean, sanitary, dry surface. The mare should be situated to help facilitate easy observation and prompt medical attention in case of an emergency.

The mare should be taken to the foaling location two to three weeks before foaling is expected to occur so that she will be comfortable in her surroundings. Research indicates that the mare produces antibodies against the pathogens in this new environment, which are then passed on to the foal in the colostrum, giving the foal passive immunity for a number of weeks after delivery.

Preparations for foaling

Long before the mare is due to foal, it is important to prepare for the birth of the foal by collecting the necessary supplies and keeping them in the stable or barn area in a covered container. To prepare the mare for parturition, you are going to need tail wrapping material

> ## Tip
> ### It was a dark and stormy night...
> Most foals are born between 10 pm and 4 am. If your foaling area lacks lighting, be prepared with a good flashlight with fresh batteries. Even if your foaling area has lighting, a flashlight may be useful in getting a better view of things.

for the mare's tail such as veterinary wrap or strips of gauze, several pairs of latex or rubber gloves, preferably sterile, and Betadine or Nolvasan solution. In addition you should have a flashlight with new and spare batteries for night time foaling or for better sight in the subdued lighting of the foaling stall or area. Most foals are born between 10 pm and 4 am, so having adequate lighting is important. Add a watch or clock for timing the mare along with your veterinarian's phone number to your supplies.

You will also need several large towels and a few hand towels, clean, sharp scissors, clamps or hemostats to control bleeding and suture thread or sterilized fishing line along with a roll of cotton, plus a large thick garbage bag for the placenta. A bucket with soap for washing hands and arms, sanitary hand wipes, plus plenty of clean, fresh water will be necessary. You will also need an enema of buffered phosphate to help pass the meconium stools of the foal.

Stages of foaling

During stage one of labor the muscles in uterine wall begin contractions and the water breaks expelling 2 to 5 gallons of fluid. Contractions continue as the muscles in the mare's abdomen begin positioning the foal for the actual birth. Once it is obvious that the birth process has begun, the mare's tail should be wrapped and the perineal area thoroughly washed.

During this first stage the mare will be restless and shifting positions. This helps position the foal in the birth canal. Once the water breaks, the mare moves into the second state of delivery. This stage may take only a few minutes or may last an hour or so. Any abnormality during the second state is an emergency. If after a few minutes' effort, two feet and a muzzle do not appear, contact the vet immediately. Normally the mare will be in a recumbent position and should begin to present a white amniotic sac.

The second stage is the actual delivery. The uterine walls contract forcefully and the mare lies down. Forceful straining of the muscles of the mare's abdomen push the foal through the birth canal, and initially, a membranous sac will appear at her vulva. The foal's leg and neck movements usually break this membrane that is called the amnion.

If the sac is velvety-red in color, it should be ruptured and the foal removed as quickly as possible. The vet should be called immediately.

It is perfectly normal for the mare to get up and down or roll, but if prolonged agitation occurs or labor exceeds two hours, an experienced individual or veterinarian should determine the best course of action.

As the head is exposed, breathing begins and within a short period of time, delivery of the hind legs and body occur. Any abnormality during the second stage of labor is an emergency. As soon as the foal's head is presented, remove fluid from the nostrils and evaluate the breathing rate of the foal. If the foal is distressed or is limp or weak, the amnion should be broken immediately and the head lifted and nostrils cleared to aid breathing. The foal is born with the umbilical cord attached and is being nurtured with the mare's blood. It is important that the cord is not severed. The cord breaks naturally as the foal moves. The mare will normally extend her neck to sniff her new foal, and it is important to give her time to begin the bonding process.

Stage three of labor is the cleaning-out stage when the placental membranes are expelled from the mare's uterus. During the third stage, the mare expels the afterbirth. It may be expelled with the foal, but if not, it is best to tie it up so that the mare won't step in it and risk breaking off pieces in the uterus. Once the placenta is delivered, it should be checked for completeness, placed in a strong plastic bag and saved for the veterinarian's examination. The placenta should always be checked carefully to determine that is has all been expelled and that no pieces have remained in the mare to cause infection.

Roughly twenty minutes after birth, the foal should be attempting to stand and then walk. It should be given a phosphate enema to ease the passage of meconium. Some foals might require two enemas, but only if necessary.

At this point the foal should be seeking the mare's udder. If he or she has trouble finding it, guiding the lip of the foal toward the nipples can be helpful. It is very important that the foal consume the colostrum within two hours after birth. The colostrum contains important antibodies to boost the foal's immune system. If the mare is unable to give milk for some reason, substitutes can be fed.

Postpartum care of mare

After a mare has foaled, careful attention should be paid to the placenta. If it is not expelled in its entirety, toxins can build up and cause inflammation and infection. Small perineal tears are not an emergency and can be taken care of later, but if there is major injury to the mare from foaling, a veterinarian should be called immediately.

As the uterus returns to its normal size, a dark chocolate-colored vaginal discharge occurs and should disappear within about a week. If the discharge is bloody, yellowish for foul-smelling or pus-like the mare should be checked for uterine infection, retained placenta or postpartum metritis. Monitor the mare's temperature for the first few days postpartum. A temperature above 101° F or 38° C indicates fever and infection.

The mare's udder should receive special attention and cleansed with warm water and ivory soap to remove secretions. In many cases, wax will develop at the tips of the mare's nipples, and they may begin to drip. If there is evidence of extended dripping,(white spots on the mares hind legs where drops have fallen), the mare should be lightly milked.

The mare should be provided with ample hay, plenty of fresh water and a warm bran mash should be fed to ease digestion through her likely bruised digestive system. A meal of mash during the next few days should also be supplied. She may be susceptible to constipation and colic as her system adjusts. To prevent these problems, her feed should be cut back by half and gradually increased over the next 10 days, and care taken to ensure that both the mare and the foal remain healthy.

Foal care

The first step after delivery is to make sure the foal is breathing. If the foal does not begin breathing on its own, tickle its nostril with a piece of straw or grass or blow into the foal's mouth to

> ## Note
> ### The mare-foal bond
>
> Directly after birth it is best to leave the mare and her foal to themselves. This is not a good time for visitors, or noisy activity. This is a time for the mother to clean the foal, and for the foal to gain coordination and begin feeding.

stimulate the respiratory reflex. Some foals require vigorous rubbing or even lifting them and dropping them from about one foot off the ground to shock the foal slightly and initiate the breathing response. Once you know the foal is breathing, it is best to leave the foaling area and observe the mare and foal from a distance.

A normal, healthy foal generally lifts its head and neck and rolls onto its chest within a few seconds of delivery. As the foal moves away from the mare the umbilical cord usually breaks. Once the umbilical cord breaks, the stump should be dipped in a mild 1 to 2 percent iodine solution. Continue to examine the naval stump for several days after birth to make sure it remains dry and doesn't become infected.

With the new foal, the time line of what to expect begins with the foal breathing within seconds. It then lifts head within 5 minutes, attempts to get up within 10 minutes, stands up usually within 30 minutes, defecates meconium within 30 minutes, vocalizes within 45 minutes, suckles for the first time within one hour, walks or runs within 90 minutes, and takes its first nap within 2 hours. Of course, this time-line is based on the average new foal, so yours may do some things more quickly or wait longer.

It usually takes some time for the foal to discover its feet and legs, and attempt to stand. If the foal does not stand within two hours, consult with your veterinarian about possible reasons for the lack of activity. It is best to let your foal begin standing and walking on its own. If you try to help it too much, the muscles, ligaments, and tendons may not be ready, and injuries may occur.

Once the new foal is able to stand, it will begin looking for the mare's udder so it can nurse. After some fumbling about and with some help from the mare, most foals will begin to nurse. This is of critical importance since the foal receives the anti-body-rich colostrum that helps protect it from disease. If the foal doesn't begin nursing within three hours, it should be checked to find out why it is not nursing.

Once the foal shows interest in nursing, you may need to help guide it to the mare's udder. You may also hand milk a few drops of colostrum from the mare and coat your fingers and the mare's teats with it. Get the foal to suck your fingers and gradually move your finger beside the mare's teat, then slowly pull your finger out of the foal's mouth and help it switch to the teat.

Use extreme caution whenever working with the foal and mare. Mares can become very protective and aggressive if they think you are a threat to their foal.

Early stages care of the mare and foal

During the first weeks of life, the mare's milk will provide all the nutrition the foal needs for sustenance. For the mare to provide the best nutrition, the mare needs almost double the amount of feed she required during pregnancy with adequate protein, vitamins and minerals, and plenty of water, not only for her own health but for the health of the foal.

> ### Note
> #### Imprinting?
>
> Some horse breeders, and even veterinarians are enthusiasts for equine imprinting. During imprinting, which takes place soon after birth, the foal is submitted to various "stimulations" with the belief that this reduces later negative or aggressive reactions. Researchers have studied this concept in detail, and generally conclude that the long-term benefits of imprinting are not sure, and some harm may result.

During this early time period, the foal's nursing habits should be observed carefully. If the foal is suckling for more than 30 minutes, it may mean that it is not getting enough milk. In this case, supplemental feed or milk replacer may be necessary for healthy development.

Twelve hours after foaling, the mare should be dewormed with Ivermectin or a product recommended by your veterinarian. Where threadworms are a problem, the foal should be treated at three weeks and begin receiving regular deworming as suggested by your veterinarian. If your veterinarian recommends it, vaccination against rhinopneumonitis and influenza can begin shortly after birth.

The foal should begin to pass meconium stools within the first 12 hours after birth. This greenish-brown to black material accumulates in the foal's intestinal tract prior to birth. By the fourth day, it will be replaced by the yellow feces of the normal foal.

Exercise, feeding, and general care

Exercise is important for both the new foal and the mare. They may be turned out as early as the first or second day after foaling takes place. Exercise should be increased gradually as weather permits. The mare and foal should be kept separated from other horses until the foal is three to four weeks old.

Resistance-free exercises include pressing down on the foal's withers and stroking the girth to get the foal used to actions and processes that will occur repeatedly later on are often suggested. Rubbing the ears and head, examining the teeth and mouth, and taking the foal's rectal temperature should be done gradually and gently with the acceptance of the mother.

Some foals show interest in feed as early as 10 to 14 days of age. As the youngster nibbles and learns to eat solid food, its digestive system adapts to the dietary changes. If the foal has diarrhea, it is important to keep the foal dry and clean around its tail and perineum. Zinc oxide may be applied to prevent scalding.

As the foal grows, its needs change, and by 8 to 10 weeks of age, mare's milk may not be sufficient to meet the foal's nutritional needs. At this point, high-quality grains and forage should be added to the foal's diet. The feed should be properly balanced for vitamins and minerals since deficits or excesses, or imbalances of needed minerals and vitamins can lead to skeletal problems. The foal should be weighed regularly and the feed quantity adjusted based on growth and fitness. A general rule to follow is one percent or a foal's body weight per day or one pound of feed per month of age. The daily ration into three or more feedings, and unlimited fresh, clean water should be available at all times.

Beginning about the third month, the mare's milk supply will gradually diminish and a natural weaning process occurs. At this time, the mare's grain should be reduced or gradually eliminated to help limit milk production, and the foal's ration should be gradually increased over a two to three week period.

Weaning the foal

Most horse handlers prefer to wean foals at five to seven months, but they may be weaned as early as four months with no adverse effects. Prior to weaning, the foal should be in good health, on a vaccination and de-worming program and eating one pound of creep ration for each month of age as well as consuming some hay or pasture. The mare is led into an adjacent pasture or paddock within sight and touch of the foal, but separated by a secure fence that won't injure the foal, but will prevent it from nursing. Although weaning is complete in one week, the mare and foal should be kept separated for approximately six weeks to prevent the mare from coming back into milk.

Conclusion

Breeding your horse, for whatever reason, requires careful thought and planning. You are responsible for the result of the breeding, and in an ethical world, your responsibility lasts as long as the life of the horse. This responsibility should be coupled with a goal of breeding a horse that is healthy, of good temperament, and genetically improved over the genetics of the mother.

In this chapter, you have been encouraged to search your soul and to think rationally about your desire to breed. There is an overpopulation of horses in the world, and the addition of more horses will only exacerbate the problem.

You have also learned about genetic conditions, and about how the selection of an appropriate stallion should be a priority. It is not necessary to spend thousands of dollars for the semen of a world champion. For most breeders, a quality local stallion may be the best choice. Pay attention to genetics and temperament of the chosen stallion. If possible, observe the offspring that have resulted from breedings with the chosen sire.

Breeding methods have advanced to improve the probability and safety of having a successful pregnancy. Discuss these methods with your veterinarian as you establish goals for the breeding. You have learned about the technologies, but should work with those experienced in breeding to make the right decision for your horse.

Lastly, you have learned the basics of foal care. The beauty of the foal and her dam running and kicking in playful activity is heart warming. The best advice is to leave the mother, and hopefully a small herd group, to care for and educate the baby for the first years of his life, but for veterinary and farrier care, you should remember the basics that you learned in this chapter. Giving your foal the proper level of contact and training while young will relate to the safety and success of your horse throughout his life.

Top-5 takeaways

The decision to breed your horse should be carefully considered. There are more horses in the world than are needed, and horse over-population affects the well being of all horses.

1. Consider the quality of your breeding animals, and always plan on improving the offspring through careful selection of the stallion.

2. Technology today allows the horse owner to widen the scope of potential stallions. Artificial insemination and embryo transfer techniques allow you to find a superior match for your mare.

3. All but an exceptional few male horses should be gelded. Stallions are unpredictable and dangerous, and should only be managed by professional horse breeders.

4. The demands of pregnancy require diet changes and attention to the potential of disease transmitted to the foal. Ask your veterinarian to provide a time line for specific treatments that should occur during pregnancy.

5. Please take responsibility for the offspring of your mare. Since you were instrumental in giving it life, you should also be responsible that the life is a good one!

Appendix A Glossary

abortion
The death and expulsion of a fetus.

abscess
A collection of pus in an area beneath the skin, in an organ, or within the body.

aerobic
Active or occurring in the presence of oxygen.

alfalfa
A perennial legume used as hay and forage.

anaerobic
Occurring without the presence of oxygen.

allergen
A substance that creates an allergic reaction.

analgesic
A pain reliever.

anaphylactic
An exaggerated reaction to a foreign protein such as that in a bee sting.

analysis
The act of testing to determine the composition and nutritional value

of hay or other feed.

anemia

A reduction of red blood cells to below a normal level.

anestrus

The stage of the estrous cycle where little ovarian activity occurs.

anhydrosis

Lacking the ability to sweat.

anthelmintic

A medication that acts to destroy intestinal parasitic worms.

antibodies

Proteins produced by the immune system to neutralize the effects of a disease-causing antigen.

antidote

A remedy to counteract the effects of poison or other harmful substances.

antivenin

An antitoxin to counteract venom, usually that from a snake or spider bite.

Arabians

A breed of swift compact horses originally developed in Arabia.

arterial

Of or relating to the artery; referring to the bright red blood present in the arteries.

arteries

The elastic-walled tubes that move blood from the heart through the body.

artificial insemination

The means of producing a pregnancy without live cover or naturally.

aspirate

To remove by suction; to take into the lungs through aspiration.

ataxia

Incoordination or the inability to move voluntary muscles that may be related to disease or injury or a nervous system disorder.

azoturia

A condition characterized by muscle cramping in the hind legs and dark-colored urine; also known as tying up.

Betadine

A microbicide used as an antiseptic and also as a scrub.

biotin

A water-souble B vitamin used in supplements to increase production of keratin, an important protein in hair and hooves.

body scoring

A numerical system used in determining body fitness.

borborygmus

The sounds produced in the horse's gut during the digestion of feed.

breeding

The act of producing offspring by mating a mare with a stallion.

breeds

Groups of horses with similar characteristics descended from common ancestors.

bruised

Characterized by an injury that causes bleeding from small blood vessels beneath the skin resutling in discoloration.

bruises

Injuries to areas beneath the skin resulting in contained bleeding and discoloration.

buckets

Containers usually with handles that are useful for carrying feed, water, and other substances.

buffered

Protected from harm by a cushion or material that prevents damage or shock.

bursa

A closed sac of fluid lined by a membrane that secretes lubricating fluid at strategic points between joints.

bursitis

A condition caused by an inflamed bursa that causes stiffness and created pain.

caballus

A predecessor of the modern horse now known as Equus Caballus.

calluses

Toughened, thickened areas of skin or other surfaces on the body.

cancer

A tumor on the surface or within the body that has the potential to destroy healthy cells and cause death.

canine

A pointed conical tooth.

canker

An erosive or spreading sore.

cannon bone

An important bone that extends from the knee or the hock to the fetlock.

canter

A 3 beat gait that is slightly slower and smoother than a gallop.

capillary

One of a system of blood vessels forming a network throughout the body.

capillary refill time

The time it takes blood to flow back into the gums after being firmly pressed with a finger; a vital sign related to circulation.

capsule

A membrane or sac enclosing a body or hoof part.

cartilage

A somewhat elastic tissue that comprises parts of the body.

cartilages

The smooth and resilient tissues that allow the ends of bones to move smoothly within joints.

castrate

To remove a horse's testicles resulting in a gelding.

cavity

A hollow place within the body; an area of tooth decay.

cementum

The bone-like tissue covering the root of a tooth within the gum.

cervix

The lower narrow part of the uterus.

charger

A horse used in the military or in parades.

chewing

The process of grinding and pulverizing feed with the teeth; masticating.

chorionic

Relating to the outer embryonic membrane known as the placenta.

circling

A locomotor stereotypy involving walking in circles in a repetitious manner.

clinchers
A farrier's tool used in shoeing horses.

clinching
The act of flattening and securing horse shoe nails.

cloning
The act of producing an organism or animal by asexually replicating cells that are genetically identical.

clover
A legume with groups of leaves and flowers grown for use as hay or forage.

coffin bone
The principle bone within the horse's hoof.

Coggins test
A test used in the diagnosis of equine infectious anemia developed by a veterinary virologist, Leroy Coggins.

cold-blood
A term describing breeds of large horses originally used for farm and draft work.

collar
A piece of tack placed around a horse's neck as part of a system for pulling a wagon or farm implement.

colic
A descriptive term referring to a group of signs that indicate abdominal pain and relate to dysfunction within the gastro-intestinal tract.

colt
A male horse younger than three years of age.

colostrum
The important first milk of the mare containing antibodies to protect the foal from diseases during its early months.

composting
The act of treating manure and vegetatitive matter so it decomposes and turns into nutrient rich fertilizer.

compound
A drug or medication made by a pharmacist by combining ingredients into a customized medication.

conformation
How the contours, angles, and shapes of the horse conform to the

breed standard; also related to the structural shape of the equine.

concussion
The force that travels vertically up a horse's leg as its hoofs hit the ground; also damage to the brain from a blow.

concussive
Related to the force that occurs when a moving hoof or object hits a hard, stationary surface causing a jarring effect.

conditioning
The use of exercise to induce physiological and structural adaptations to maximize performance and maintain soundness.

congenital
Originating from birth or or acquired during development in the uterus.

cool-down
Taking action to bring a horse's temperature back into the normal range after exercise or on a hot day.

coprophagy
The act of eating manure or dirt.

corium
The dermo-epidermal layer containing many small blood vessels situated between the coffin bonetween the hoof wall.

coronary band
A thick band of vascular tissue in the coronet of the horse's hoof.

creep feed
Supplemental feed given to foals before weaning.

cribbing
A stereotypy evidenced by a horse grasping a solid object such as a fence rail with its teeth while gulping air.

cruciate ligament
Either of two ligaments in the horse's leg that cross each other from femur to tibia.

cushion
A fibrous padding that serves as protection between body or hoof parts.

cystitis
Inflammation of the urinary bladder.

deciduous
Early teeth or milk teeth that are shed at a certain stage of growth;

also plants and trees that shed their leaves.

dentin

The hard material that composes most of a tooth.

detoxified

Having a harmful substance removed or neutralized so it no longer affects the body.

detraining

The sudden cessation of training with a resultant loss in fitness.

diagnostic

The use of methods and tests leading to a diagnosis.

diarrhea

A condition where the manure is loose, watery, and frequent and with an increase in the amount expelled.

digital

Providing a read out in numerical figures; done with a finger as in a rectal examination.

disease

A condition in the animal that impairs normal function and presents with symptoms of illness.

dissecans

Related to the separation of immature joint cartilege from the under-lying bone.

dominance

Related to functional asymmetry of parts of the body with one side being stronger; showing stronger control in a situation.

dynamic

Related to active movement in exercise to increase suppleness and strength as in moving a joint or limb through a range of motion.

dysplasia

Abnormal anatomical structure related to growth as in knock knees or bow legs.

dyspnea

Inability to breath properly; difficult or labored respiration.

electrolytes

Minerals necessary for organ functions usually given in water in con-juntion with exercise to replenish body fluids.

embryo

An animal in the early stages of growth within the uterus before organ development begins.

endorphins

Brain chemicals released during exercise that create a positive feeling within the body; peptides released in the brain having a pharmacological effect.

endotoxins

Toxins that are part of the outer cell wall of bacteria and are released when the cell is ruptured.

enzymes

Complex proteins that catalyze bio-chemical reactions such as in the digestive process as feed is broken down.

equine

Any horse or horse-like animal, especially one of the genus Equus.

esophagus

A muscular tube that begins at the back of the mouth and passes through the neck into the top of the stomach.

estrous

Related to the reproductive cycle as determined by times of ovulation.

estrus

Heat; the phase of the estrous cycle during which the mare is receptive to the stallion.

euphoric

Having a heightened sense of well-being or elation.

exercises

Activities related to bodily exertion to develop and maintain physical strength and fitness.

exertional

Related to vigorous physical action; also relates to a state of immobility when muscle masses disrupt during exercise.

fallopian tube

The tube that carries the egg from the ovary to the uterus.

farrier

A specialist in hoof care including trimming, balancing, and shoeing.

fetus

The developing organism older than 14 days usually after organ development begins.

fescue

A type of grass often used as hay and forage.

filly

A young female horse less than three years old.

fetlock

A part of the horse's leg formed by the joint between the cannon bone and the pastern bone. Also, the tuft of hair on the projection.

fistula

An abnormal connection between two body parts usually occurring because of injury or surgery.

fitness

The state of physical condition and and how it relates to requirements for performance at increasing levels.

flares

Related to the outward bending of the hoof wall; also a stretched whiteline where the hoof wall separates fro the coffin bone.

flexion

A bending movement engaging a joint in a limb.

floating

The process of rasping or filing a horse's teeth to limit growth and maintain chewing surfaces.

foal

A young horse less than four months old.

follicle

A growth within the ovary that contains an egg; also the cells within the skin from which hairs grow.

forage

To wander in search of food; to graze or browse; feed for horses such as hay and grasses.

forages

Feed for horses including hay, grass, and other suitable plant material.

founder

Also known as laminitis, a condition tht occurs in the feet leading to lameness and is sometimes caused by overfeeding.

fracture

A break in a bone.

gallop

A fast natural 3 beat gait of a horse.

gamete

A mature male or female germ cell usually containing a set of chromosones.

gastric

Related to the the stomach.

gelding

A male horse that has been castrated.

genetics

The science related to genes, the origin, and development of inherited traits based on genetic makeup.

gestation

The period of time when the developing young are carried in the uterus; pregnancy.

glycogen

The principle form in which glucose is is stored in animal tissue.

groundwork

Basic exercises for horses often in an arena or pen used to teach, train, and condition the horse.

hardeners

Special treatments for hooves that increase the strength and hardness of the hoof wall.

heat

Also known as estrus: The period of time when the mare is receptive to the stallion.

Henneke

A system of evaluating a horse's condition on a numerical scale originated by Dr. Henneke and colleagues at Texas A&M University.

herbivore

One of the group of mammals that depends on plants for nutrition.

hierarchy

The established social system within a group of animals.

hind-gut

The part of the horse's digestive system that includes the intestine where fermentation to break down cellulose takes place

hoof tester

An instrument shaped like a pair of pincers used to squeeze parts of the hoof to determine areas of pain indicating abscesses and other problems.

hormones

Products of living cells that circulate in the body and produce stimulatory effects.

horseshoe

A covering for the bottom of a horse's hoof usually made of metal.

hyaluronic

Related to a viscous polysaccharide with lubricating properties present in the synovial fluid in joints.

imaging

The process of creating visual representations of the interior of the body for clinical analysis and medical intervention.

immunity

A condition of being able to resist a particular disease by counteracting its effects.

impaction

The state of having a blockage in the throat or digestive system that impedes normal workings of the system.

incisors

The cutting teeth located between the canine teeth.

incumbent

A state of lying down; unable to get up.

infection

A disease or sore caused by a bacteria, fungus, or virus.

influenza

A severe respiratory disease marked by fever, prostration, severe aches and pains and inflammation of respiratory membranes.

injury

A wound or trauma caused by an external force.

insulin

A natural hormone made by the pancreas that controls the level of sugar glucose in the blood.

intubation

The process of putting a tube in place in a hollow part of the body such as the trachea or the stomach as part of a medical intervention.

ivermectin

A drug mixture used in veterinary medicine as a deworming agent.

jaundice

A condition leading to a yellowing of the skin and eyes caused by bile pigments.

joints

The points of contact within the musculoskeletal parts of the anatomy where bones meet in a system that allows movement.

keratin

The fibrous proteins that make up horny epidermal tissues such as hair and hoof walls.

keratoma

An area of hardened skin usually called a callus.

kicking

Striking outward with the hooves and legs.

laceration

A cut or injury that goes through the skin into the flesh.

lactate

Secrete milk.

lactic

Involving the production of lactic acid, a compound formed in the body in anaerobic metabolism of a carbohydrate and also produced by bacerial action in milk.

lamellae

A thin plate, scale, or membrane as of bone, tissue or cell walls.

laminitis

Inflammation of sensitive laminae in the hoof of a horse caused by stressful events, trauma, or over feeding; also known as founder.

lateral

Situated on, directed to, or coming from the side.

legume

An important feed and forage group of plants that are used as hay such as clover and alfalfa.

ligaments

Bands of fibrous tissue connecting bones and cartilages serving to strengthen and support joints.

linear

Of or relating to a straight line.

loading

Manipulation of diet and exercise to increase muscle, blood flow, respiration, and other factors related to improvement in performance.

locomotor

Related to the systems that produce movement through use of the limbs and body.

longeing
A technique for exercising horses where a horse is worked on a line/rope and respond to the commands of a handler or trainer.

lysine
A basic amino acid that is a constituent of most proteins and is an essential nutrient in the diet of horses.

mare
A mature female horse over three years of age.

masticate
To chew or pulverize with the teeth.

maxillary
Related to the two bones that are in the upper jaw and used for chewing.

meconium
The dark greenish mass that accumulates in the bowel during fetal life and is expelled after foaling.

membranes
The thin, pliable layer of soft covering on a body part that helps protect and maintain it.

meniscal
A fibrous cartilage within a joint, especially the knee.

metabolic
Related to or based on metabolism by which energy is provided for vital processes.

methionine
A naturally occuring amino acid necessary for normal metabolism.

muscle
Tissue composed of fibers and cells that have the ability to contract producing movement in the body; an organ composed of muscle tissue.

myoglobin
An iron-containing protein found in muscle fibers having a high affinity for oxygen.

myopathy
Any abnormality or disease of muscle tissue.

navicular
Related to the navicular bone in the feet of the horse and the soft tissue structure that comprises the navicular apparatus.

neonatal

Relating to and affecting the newborn foal.

Nolvasan

A disinfectant for equine wounds; also used s a surgical scrub

NSAIDs

Any of the nonsteroidal anti-inflammatory drugs used in the horse including aspirin, diclofenac sodium, ketoprofen, phenylbutazone, etc.

orthopedic

Related to the correction and treatment of bone disorders and diseases.

osselets

A condition affecting the front fetlock joint caused by stress or injury from repeated concussive forces.

osteitis

Inflammation of a bone.

ovulation

The process during which the egg follicle releases the egg into the oviduct.

oxidative

Related to the process of dehydrognization using the action of oxygen.

palmar

The term used when referring to particular structures of the forelimb of the horse.

palpation

The act of examining by touch with a probing movement.

papillae

Any of protrusion of a body part such as a nipple; a connective tissue that nourishes the hair or a developing tooth; the taste buds.

parasite

An organism that lives on or within another organism and depends on it for its existence without giving anything in return.

passive

Related to a form of exercise that relies on external force for movement and development.

pasterns

The part of the foot of the horse that extends from the fetlock to the top of the hoof.

pasture

An area devoted to plants for feeding grazing animals.

pathogen

A specific causitive agent such as a bacteria or virus that causes a disease.

pawing

The act of scraping or beating at the ground with the hoof.

perineum

An outer area of tissue that marks externally the boundary of the outlet of the pelvis and gives passage to the external genitalia.

phosphate

An organic compound that permits useful energy to be released through metabolism

physeal

Relating to the area of bone that separates the metaphysis and the epiphysis in which the cartilage grows.

physiology

The branch of biology that deals with the functions of life or living matter such as cells, organs, and tissues.

picking

The act of using a tool to remove dirt, gravel and debris from a horse's hoofs.

pituitary

A small endocrine organ that releases secretions that affect most basic body functions.

placenta

The vascular organ in animals that unites the fetus to the uterus and provides nourishment to the developing animal.

plasma

The fluid part of blood.

platelet

A minute disk-like part of mammalian blood that assists in clotting of the blood.

postpartum

Occurring in or during the period following parturition; following giving birth.

poultices

A medicated substance spread on cloth and applied to sores, lesions, or a part of the body affected by a disease; such as on the chest.

prebiotic

Non-digestible food ingredients that promote the growth of beneficial microorganisms in the intestines.

pregnancy

The condition of containing a growing embryo, fetus orunborn offspring within the body.

premolars

Teeth situated in front of or preceding the molar teeth.

probiotics

Microorganisms introduced into the body for healthful effects usually a dairy food or a supplement containing live bacteria.

processed

Relating to grain or other feed that has been changed in form from its natural state.

protein

Any of the naturally occurring complex substances composed of chains of amino acids that are an essential part of living organisms.

protozoa

A diverse group of single-celled organisms that can divide only within a host organism and cause diseases such as malaria.

puncture

A hole or wound caused by the penetration of a hard object.

quittor

A purulent inflammation of the feet of equines characterized by chronic inflammation and the formation of fitulas opening above the coronet.

rabies

An acute viral disease that affects the nervous system usually the result of an animal affected by the disease.

ration

The amount of feed given to a particular animal during the day.

receptor

Cells that are capable of responding to an external stimulus and transmits a signal to a sensory nerve.

rectal

Related to the terminal part of the intestine, the rectum.

refill time

Related to the time it takes for color to return to an external capillary that has been pressed upon.

reinforcer

A signal or reward that is used in training a horse once the horse accomplishes a given task.

resistance

Of or relating to exercise involving pushing or working against a source of resistance such as a weight to increase strength.

resonance imaging

Related to imaging of the foot or a part of the body with magnetic resonance imaging.

restraints

Methods to secure a horse while working on or with it such as tack, a twitch, a tie-down or a chemical.

retained

Kept within the body such as milk teeth that remain after other teeth are present, or a body part such as an undescended testicle.

retina

The sensory membrane that lines the eye and functions as the source of vision by receiving an image and transmitting it to the brain.

roughage

Food that contains indigestible material acting as fiber.

ruptured

The state of being broken apart as in the case of severe tissue damage that exposes inside of the organ or bone.

saline solution

Containing a salt such as potassium or sodium that has a carthartic action; or a salt solution that is isotonic with blood used in medicine.

schooling

The process of exercising and training a horse for service or in the formal techniques of equitation.

secretions

A product of a gland or organ that serves a useful function such as saliva to aid in digestion.

sedation

Inducing a calm, tranquilized, state through the use of a sedative.

selenium

A trace mineral vital for proper muscle development.

sensory
Related to the nerve impulses from the sensory organs to nerve centers creating awareness of sights, sounds, odors, etc.

sesamoid
A bone embedded in a tendon; a nodular mass of bone such as the patella or cartilage in a tendon.

sheared
Having a distortion especially in the hoof capsule leading to structural breakdown as in sheared heels.

sheath
The tubular fold of skin covering the penis.

shoeing
The process of fitting and placing ametal rim or covering on the bottom of a horse's hoof.

sidebones
An orthopedic condition in horses that occurs when the co-lateral cartilage within the hoof ossifies resulting in lameness.

sinuses
The narrow elongated tracts that allow secretions such as mucous or pus to drain through a nostril or other opening.

sinusitis
A condition where the sinuses become inflamed.

slurry
A mixture of a powdered substance such as charcoal with water used to purge poison or other harmful substances from the horse's digestive tract.

smooth mouth
When a horse's molars are worn so that dentine and enamel are evenly worn making thorough chewing difficult.

solution
A combination of ingredients thoroughly mixed with water or other liquid such as an antiseptic to be used as a wound treatment.

spavin
A bony enlargement of the hock of a horse associated with strain.

speculum
An instrument inserted into the horse's mouth to hold it open and allow visual inspection and dental care.

splint

A bony enlargement on the upper part of the cannon bone usually on the inside of the leg.

splints

A thin piece of wood or other rigid material used to immobilize a fractured or dislocated bone.

sprain

A tearing of fibrous tissue such as a muscle, ligament, or joint capsule caused by forced movement beyond the normal range.

stallion

A mature male horse that has not been castrated and is usually used for breeding.

stifle

The joint above the hock in the hind leg.

stomach

The organ within the body where feed is held and digested.

strains

Stretched, torn or over-used muscles or tendons characterized by painful swelling accompanied by lameness.

stress

A state of bodily or mental tension resulting from factors that cause pressure on an organism.

stringhalt

A gait problem that causes a horse to lift his legs higher and more rapidly than usual resulting in a lack of control.

sucking

Drawing in through the mouth as in a foal nursing or a horse engaged in cribbing or wind sucking.

Sudangrass

A vigorously growing annual sorgham grass used for hay and forage.

sulfate

A salt or ester of sulfuric acid used in medications.

suppling

The process of using exercises to increase joint range of motion to help the horse move smoothly and athletically.

surgery

A branch of medicine relate to operative procedures to correct physical problems.

suspensory

Related to the fibrous membranes that support and suspend an organ or body part such as the suspensory ligaments in the limbs.

sutures

Stitches used to close a wound or cut.

syndrome

A group of signs or symptoms that occur together and characterize an abnormality or condition.

system

Any of the connected interacting or interdependent parts of the body unified as a whole such as the respiratory system.

tailhead

The beginning of the tail where the tail joins the rump.

tartar

An encrustation on the teeth consisting of plaque hardened by mineral salts.

tendon

A tough cord or band of fibrous connective tissue that unites a muscle and another part such as a bone to transmit force into movement.

tendonitis

Inflammation of a tendon.

tetanus

An acute infectious disease caused by an endotoxin of a bacterium usually introduced through a wound.

thrush

An infection in the hoofs caused by a fungus characterized by a foul-smelling discharge.

toed-out

Having a conformation defect where the toes point outward resulting in a splay footed way of moving forward.

tomography

A method of producing a three dimensional image of the internal structures of the body and/or the limbs.

topical

Applied to the skin or other surface of the body usually to aid in healing or protecting the area.

toxins

Poisonous substances that are specific products of metabolic processes of a living organism and are usually very toxic.

turnout

Putting a horse in a pasture or other area where he can engage in free physical activity.

twitch

A device used to control a horse usually a chain or rope in such a way as to calm and restrain a horse during a procedure.

tying-up

A muscle metabolism problem that causes stiffness and soreness leading to a reluctance to move; also known as azoturia and exertional rhabdomyolysis.

ultrasound

The diagnostic use of a noninvasive imaging technique for examining the interior of the body.

uterine

Having to do with the uterus, the muscular organ for containing and nourishing the developing fetus.

vascular

Related to the blood vessel system of the body.

warm-up

The process of slowly getting the horse's body ready for more vigorous exercise and activity.

weaning

The process of changing over from nursing by the mare to eating hay and grain as a regular diet.

weanlings

Foals that are newly weaned around 5 to 7 months old.

weaving

A locomotor stereotypy involving horse weaving its head and neck rhythmically either while walking or standing still.

whiteline

The juncture between the laminae and the inner hoof wall in the horse's hoof.

withers

The area between the shoulder bones of the horse.

wobblers

A condition that affects the gait of a horse when growth abnormalities or joint arthritis put pressure on the spinal cord causing an ataxic gait.

wounds

Injuries that cause a breaking or lacerating of the skin resulting in damage to the underlying tissue or bone.

yearlings

Young horses that have reached the age of one year.

Appendix B References

Books

Horse Genetics

A classic for horse breeders. Covers in detail the genetic components of many horse attributes, including coloration and genetic diseases and conditions.

Ann T. Bowling, *Horse Genetics*, Cambridge: CABI Publishing, 1996

Essential Principles of Horseshoeing

For the serious student of horseshoeing principles and techniques, this book is a standard for farriers worldwide. Doug Butler, Ph.D., also is a contributor to EquiMed.

Doug Butler, Jacob Butler and Peter Butler, *Essential Principles of Horseshoeing*, Crawford: Doug Butler Enterprises, Inc., 2012

Lameness - Recognizing and Treating the Horse's Most Common Ailment

A very comprehensive analysis of the various causes of lameness, along with methods of diagnosis and treatment. This book is suitable for veterinarians and those interested in a full understanding of lameness.

Christine King and Richard Mansmann, *Lameness - Recognizing and Treating the Horse's Most Common Ailment*, Guilford: The Lyons Press, 1997

The Horse Conformation Handbook

Heather Thomas, an EquiMed contributor, provides a detailed and comprehensive view of horse conformation in this wonderfully illustrated book.

Heather Smith Thomas, *The Horse Conformation Handbook*, New York: Storey Publishing, 2005

Conditioning Sport Horses

This book provides the details behind horse physiology and biology as it relates to fitness and conditioning. Hilary Clayton, DVM an EquiMed contributor, was the McPhail Dressage Chair in Equine Sports Medicine in the College of Veterinary Medicine at Michigan State University.

Hilary M. Clayton, *Conditioning Sport Horses*, Mason: Sport Horse Publications, 1991

Horse Owner's Veterinary Handbook

A long standing favorite, and deserving of a place on the book shelves of all horse owners, this veterinary handbook provides comprehensive information about equine health pertaining to veterinary medicine.

James M. Giffin and Tom Gore, *Horse Owner's Veterinary Handbook*, Second Edition, Hoboken: Wiley Publishing Inc., 1989

Feed Your Horse Like a Horse

Dr. Getty, a popular speaker and academician regarding equine nutrition, authored this comprehensive and highly interesting book dealing with horse nutrition. Juliet Getty, Ph.D., is an EquiMed contributor and strong advocate of free-choice feeding.

Juliet M. Getty, *Feed Your Horse Like a Horse*, Indianapolis: Dog Ear Publishing, 2010

Equine Dentistry: A Practical Guide

This academic treatise was written for the equine dental care practitioner in mind.

Patricia Pence, Equine Dentistry: A Practical Guide, Baltimore: Lippencott Williams & Wilkins, 2002

Groom to Win

One of author Mark Sellers' favorite books. Susan Harris covers more than grooming in this well written and very informative book. If you show horses, or care about maintaining a healthy and beautiful horse, this book is a must read.

Susan E. Harris, *Groom to Win*, Second Edition, New York: Wiley Publishing, Inc., 1991

Humane Livestock Handling

Not a horse book per se, but Temple Grandin provides unique insight into how all prey animals think and perceive their surroundings. Much of the current ideas behind horse handling are explained in this accessible volume.

Temple Grandin, *Humane Livestock Handling*, North Adams: Storey Publishing, 2008

Equine Behavior - A Guide for Veterinarians and Equine Scientists

Paul McGreevy, Ph.D. wrote this book for practitioners of veterinary medicine as a comprehensive and researched guide to equine behavior. Particularly interesting are the chapters devoted to perception and learning.

Paul McGreevy, *Equine Behavior - A Guide for Veterinarians and Equine Scientists*, Second Edition, Sydney: Saunders Elsevier, 2012.

Websites

EquiMed.com

A comprehensive website about horse health. The authors of this book are founders and editors of this website.

Horse-Health-Matters.com

A website dedicated to this book. You will find the author's blog, errata, web tools, videos, calculators and more. This is also the website where you can purchase Horse Health Matters and related books by EquiMed Press.

thehorse.com

The oldest website and magazine that addresses equine health. Thousands of articles are available online covering a wide variety of equine related health issues.

Appendix C Horse Math

How much does my horse weigh?

Knowing your horse's weight is needed for two primary health related issues: 1) how much to feed your horse; and 2) how much medication do you administer to your horse.

Unfortunately, horses are too heavy to easily weight on a scale. If you have access to a livestock scale, you are in luck - no math required! If you don't have access to a scale, measuring and calculating your horse's weight is quite simple.

Basic measurement

You will need two pieces of baling twine, a pair of scissors, a tape measure and a calculator. You will use the twine to more safely measure the circumference of the horse's body at the withers and the horse's body length. First, take one piece of twine and tie a single knot it it. This piece of twine will be used to measure the heart girth. Take the twine and drape it over the withers. Safely reach under your horse's girth, and

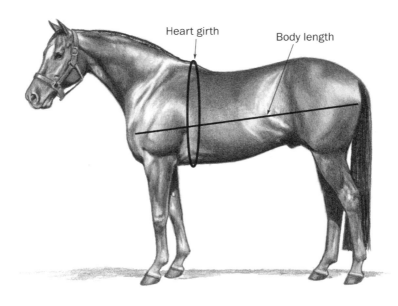

Heart girth

Body length

bring the twine together snuggly. Using your scissors, cut the twine in the area of overlap. The piece from around the body is the same length as the horse's heart girth.

Take the second piece of twine and tie two knots in it. Stand facing your horse and with your left hand, feel for the point of the shoulder. Start in the middle of the chest, and move toward the shoulder until you feel the bone joint. This joint is relatively easy to find. See the illustration of the horse above to better visualize what you are feeling. With your right hand, find the point of buttocks. The point of buttocks is on the rear of the horse normally about four inches below the tail and slightly off to the side. Once again, refer to the illustration to visualize what you are trying to locate. The point of buttock may be more difficult to feel, but get as close as possible.

Now, using the twine with two knots, measure between these two points. Depending on the size of your horse and your arm span, you may need help to do this. Cut this piece of twine to the length between these two points.

Next, measure the length of the two twines using your tape measure. Measure in inches or centimeters. Note the length of the twine with one knot is the heart girth (HG). Write this down. Note the length of the twine with two knots is the body length (BL). Write this down.

Using your calculator, calculate your horse's weight using the following formula:

If you measured in inches

Weight in pounds = (HG x HG x BL)/5389

If you measured in centimeters

Weight in kilograms = (HG x HG x BL)/11880

These formulas provide a good estimation of your horse's weight, but they assume a typical horse body form. While this estimation is adequate for feeding and most medication purposes, it is not as good as using a calibrated livestock scale.

How much should I feed my horse?

A good starting point to determine how much you should feed your horse is to use the horse's weight (HW) as a guide. Depending on the horse's use and metabolism, start with feeding 2% of the horse's weight daily, ideally spread between three feedings or even free choice.

Here is the simple formula:

Daily hay ration = HW x 0.02

If the weight is in pounds, the hay ration will be in pounds. If the weight is in kilograms, the hay ration will be in kilograms.

For example, if your horse's weight is calculated to be 1096 pounds, take 1096 times 0.02 for a daily hay ration of 22 lbs.

Remember that if your horse has a high activity level, or if your horse has a nervous temperament, you will need to feed more. If your horse is only rarely ridden, and is on not very active by nature, you will need to feed less. Also remember that a horse may be unwilling to consume enough hay to maintain weight, in which case you may need to feed grain or a weight supplement. If your horse is putting on weight (measure him from time to time), then you will need to reduce the ration.

The very best way to decide if your feeding program is on track is to body score your horse. Learn how to do this in Chapter 9.

Lastly - there is no nutritionally perfect hay. Always keep a salt/mineral block available, and discuss vitamin deficiencies that may be particular to your area or choice of hay with your veterinarian.

How much medicine does my horse need?

Again, the weight of your horse is the key factor in determining the dosage of many medications. For prescription medications, follow the prescription instructions. These are provided by the veterinarian based on the need of your animal. For non prescription medications, follow the instructions on the label. If the instructions provide for a weight dependent dose, you can mutliply your horse's weight by the dose rate to get the amount needed.

For example, if a medication indicates to feed 1 ounce per 250 pounds and your horse weighs 1096 pounds, you would calculate the amount in ounces using the following formula:

$$\text{Amount in ounces} = \text{HW x dose per pound}$$
$$= 1096 \text{ lbs x (1 ounce/250 lbs)}$$
$$= 4.4 \text{ ounces}$$

Similarly, if a medication indicates to feed 30 g per 100 kg, and your horse weighs 500 kg, you would calculate the amount in grams using the following formula:

Amount in grams $\quad$ = HW x dose per kilogram

$\qquad$ = 500 kg x (30 g/100 kg)

$\qquad$ = 150 g

If something seems to not be right, it probably isn't. For example, if the dose calculation indicates that you need to administer 4 pounds of medication, then there is probably something wrong! When in doubt, contact your veterinarian for assistance in getting the correct dose of any medication, prescription or not.

How tall is my horse?

Horses are traditionally measured in hands. The distance measured is vertical line from the top of the withers to the ground. One hand equals 4 inches or 9.8 cm. Conversion between feet-inches and hands is ease. Use the following formula:

Hands = ((feet x 12) + inches)/4

For example, say you measure from the withers to the ground and get 5 feet 10 inches. Applying the formula:

Hands = ((5 x 12) + 10)/4

$\qquad$ = (60 + 10)/4

$\qquad$ = (70/4) = 17.5 hands - a handsomely tall horse

Online resources

The internet is a great resource for assistance with simple but important math. You can find online calculators for horse weight (you still need to measure your horse), horse feeding, and dosage. We recommend the following URLs:

http://equimed.com/health-centers/equine-weight-calculator

http://equimed.com/health-centers/equine-feed-calculator

http://equimed.com/drugs-and-medications/dosage-calculator

Index